CLINICAL MANAGEMENT OF CHILDHOOD STUTTERING

CLINICAL MANAGEMENT OF CHILDHOOD STUTTERING

by
Meryl J. Wall, Ph.D.
and
Florence L. Myers, Ph.D.
Associate Professors
Department of Speech Arts and Communicative Disorders
Adelphi University

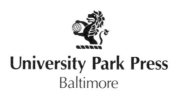

University Park Press
Baltimore

University Park Press
International Publishers in Medicine and Human Services
300 North Charles Street
Baltimore, Maryland 21201

Copyright © 1984 by University Park Press

Typeset by The TypeWorks
Manufactured in the United States of America by The Maple Press Company
Design by S. Stoneham, Studio 1812, Baltimore

Library of Congress Cataloging in Publication Data

Wall, Meryl J.
Clinical Management of Childhood Stuttering.

Includes index.
1. Stuttering in children. I. Myers, Florence L. II. Title. [DNLM:
1. Stuttering—In infancy and childhood. 2. Stuttering—Therapy.
WM 475 W187c]
RJ496.S8W35   1984   618.92′8554   84-2266
ISBN 0-8391-1883-X

Contents

Preface

Stuttering most frequently begins during childhood. Thus to prevent the normal nonfluencies of early childhood from becoming pathological, to prevent abnormal disfluencies from becoming more severe, and to develop appropriate clinical approaches for young disfluent children, we must gain a better understanding of the dynamics of childhood disfluency.

Historically more attention has been given in the literature to the confirmed older stutterer than to the young stutterer. Because there is some degree of nonfluency in children's speech during normal speech and language development, a young disfluent child often presents clinicians and parents with a twofold dilemma. First, clinicians and parents are unsure how to approach the young disfluent child. Should the disfluencies be ignored in the hope that the child will outgrow them, or should the disfluencies be dealt with directly by alleviating the symptoms? Second, the differentiation between normal and abnormal disfluency has not been clearly delineated. For example, are the fluency disruptions in normal children quantitatively or qualitatively different from those of stutterers? Should assessment and treatment of childhood stuttering consider developmental aspects of fluency behavior in children, including such variables as syllable rate, utterance length, and phoneme duration (Starkweather, 1980)?

Some scholars, such as Bloodstein (1970), place normal and abnormal disfluencies on a continuum, so that stuttering is viewed primarily as an intensification of the relatively mild and innocuous fragmentations of speech that occur during normal childhood. Other scholars, such as Wingate (1976), point toward some intrinsic and qualitative difference between normal and abnormal disruptions in the fluency of speech. The issue of whether the normal disruptions in the flow of children's speech should be viewed dichotomously from or continuously with stuttering is explored in Chapter 6.

Chapter 1 introduces the topic of childhood stuttering, including a three-factor model that provides the organizational framework for the book as well as for our assessment and therapy approach. The theories and symptomatologies of stuttering are discussed in Chapters 2 and 3, respectively. Psycholinguistic and physiological aspects of childhood stuttering are treated in Chapters 4 and 5, respectively. Chapter 6 delineates assessment approaches, and Chapters 7 and 8, respectively, summarize representative therapy approaches and discuss our own therapy approach and techniques for the clinical management of the child stutterer.

Spurred by advances in research paradigms, more research on the young disfluent child has occurred in the past few years. Research using current language sampling techniques, for example, has afforded us the opportunity for a detailed examination of the interaction between fluency and language behaviors in children. Developments on the theoretical front have also given us a more enlightened framework from which to conduct research and therapy for the disfluent child. This book discusses these new research paradigms and applies them clinically, using our three-factor model (Myers and Wall, 1982).

This book is written for advanced undergraduate and graduate students in communication disorders. Because of its emphasis on the assessment and therapeutic management of young stutterers, it also is a useful reference for practicing speech-language pathologists in schools, clinics, and hospitals. It can provide insight to allied professionals such as teachers, counselors, nurses, and physicians who encounter young disfluent children.

In preparing this text, we have been assisted in a variety of ways by many people. We particularly thank Dr. C. Woodruff Starkweather, of Temple University, who gave us invaluable help with his critique of the text. We also thank the graduate students at Adelphi University, who have so capably carried out the therapy for the cases discussed and whose shared insights assisted us in our writing. Further appreciation is extended to David Ling, who prepared the original illustration for the three-factor model.

REFERENCES

Bloodstein, O. 1970. Stuttering and normal nonfluency—A continuity hypothesis. Bri. J. Disord. Commun. 5:30–39.

Myers, F., and Wall, M. 1982. Toward an integrated approach to early childhood stuttering. J. Fluency Disord. 7:47–54.

Starkweather, C. 1980. Speech fluency and its development in normal children. In: N. Lass (ed.), Speech and Language: Advances in Basic Research and Practice, pp. 143–200, Vol. 4. Academic Press, New York.

Wingate, M. 1976. Stuttering: Theory and Treatment. John Wiley & Sons, New York.

To Elizabeth
and to the memory of
Margaret and William Johnson
M.J.W.

To my parents,
Rufus and Alice Ling,
and my husband Russell
F.L.M.

CLINICAL MANAGEMENT OF CHILDHOOD STUTTERING

1
Introduction

ATTRIBUTES OF THE MATURE
CLINICIAN TREATING THE YOUNG STUTTERER

In *The Treatment of Stuttering* (1973), Charles Van Riper reflected on the awesome task of clinicians who conduct stuttering therapy by quoting Wendell Johnson:

> *The longer I work with stutterers, the more tolerant I become of anyone who has any therapeutic ideas at all concerning it. . . . There is no such thing as the method for treating stuttering, and the fact that so many differing methods are more or less successful is of more than incidental interest*
> (Johnson, 1939, p. 170).

Van Riper and Johnson are among the most influential thinkers in the field of stuttering, and yet they along with other master clinicians approach the phenomenon with great humility. There is a lesson here for us. We should be wary of promises of a "quick cure" for stuttering. Although great advances have taken place on the theoretical and research fronts within the past decade, there has yet to be developed a single therapy program that exhaustively provides a one-to-one correspondence between the multitude of research findings and their respective applications to therapy. Clinicians should nonetheless approach the problem of stuttering with perseverance and open-mindedness. The mature clinician treating childhood stuttering should have the characteristics described in the sections that follow.

Adopting a Broadly Based View of Stuttering

Stuttering is a complex, multidimensional phenomenon. The clinician must be aware of the immensely intricate interrelation between respiration, phonation, and coarticulation—the substrata of the speech production system that are particularly relevant to fluency. Van Riper (1973) repeatedly refers to stuttering as a disorder of timing. That is, temporal disruptions of the motor patterns of syllables and words comprise the core of stuttering. Any deficit in one of these substrata of speech production, such as excessive laryngeal tension at the phonatory level, can trigger a disruption in the temporal ordering of syllables. Moreover, any deficit in the coupling of two or more of the substrata can also lead to impaired fluency. For example, the severe reduction of air supply during expiration may trigger laryngeal tension and discoordination, leading to disruptions in the normal flow of speech.

Although a great deal of emphasis has been placed on the speech production aspects of fluency and disfluency, only relatively recently has the interrelation between language and stuttering during early childhood been studied systematically. That language development itself is an enormous undertaking during childhood cannot be denied. Phonological, syntactic, semantic, and pragmatic development are all occurring at a feverish pace during the very period that the speech production system is maturing. The interplay between speech, language, and fluency development during childhood becomes increasingly synergistic with time. That is, the variables interact increasingly as the child matures during those critical early years of development. It would be wise, therefore, to view the child as a system with subcomponents that influence one another.

We propose that the clinician take a broadly based view of the young disfluent child by considering the psychosocial, physiological, and psycholinguistic variables that affect the child's disfluencies.

Cultivating Keen Observational Skills

It is no simple matter to adopt an eclectic approach in clinical practice. Because stuttering is a highly complex and multifaceted phenomenon, we must develop astute observational skills by enriching our knowledge about the factors that influence stuttering. This book aims to synthesize recent research findings and to provide for clinicians a matrix or profile of behaviors to look for when assessing or treating the young disfluent child. Undoubtedly the recent emphasis on behavior modification, particularly in vogue during the 1960s and early 1970s, has brought forth a generation of clinicians who are quite accustomed to writing behavioral objectives and specifying in detail observable behaviors. Because the state of the art is such that we cannot usually pinpoint a specific etiology for a particular stutterer, it is imperative that we be rigorous and exhaustive in our observations and descriptions of the stuttering behaviors of our clients.

Observations of stuttering behavior should be reliable and valid, acknowledging inconsistencies when they occur, while attempting to sort out patterns among apparent inconsistencies. Such observations should make allowances for inter- and intrapersonal differences when they occur. A great deal of attention has been paid in the recent literature to individual differences in children's fluency behavior, even with the early fluency disruptions of normally speaking 2-year-old children (Yairi, 1981). No longer do we hold the naive viewpoint that behavior is rigorously invariant, even for a given child at a given time. Astute observation, in summary, should view the young disfluent child from a comprehensive perspective.

Appreciating Theory and Research To Enrich Clinical Skills

Quite understandably, students often prefer to learn about the practical rather than the theoretical. At a superficial level, it is the practical information that provides great mileage in the therapy room. Looking beyond the superficial level, however, the seasoned student and the clinician find that even greater mileage is to be gained from theoretical insights and knowledge of research findings on a problem. It is from a fertile theory that significant research is generated. In turn, it is from research data that clinical strategies are drawn.

A frequent question directed to student clinicians by their supervisors is, What is the rationale for using this technique or approach? A rationale for a therapy approach often stems from the clinician's theoretical orientation to a problem. If the individual's orientation to stuttering is grounded in the viewpoint that disfluencies stem from hyperactivity and asynchrony of the laryngeal mechanism, for example, then the therapy approach selected is likely to incorporate techniques such as the use of easy onset for the initiation of syllables.

The relation between theory and practice is not unidirectional. Greater clinical experience feeds into a richer theoretical understanding of a problem by advancing hypotheses about the problem. Such hypotheses serve as the backbone of further research and theory. Wherever possible, therefore, this book integrates theory, research, and clinical endeavors to provide the reader not only "practical" suggestions for therapy but also a rationale supporting the therapeutic procedures.

Developing an Eclectic View

To be eclectic is to select "what appears to be best in various doctrines, methods, or styles . . . composed of elements drawn from various sources" (*Webster's Seventh New Collegiate Dictionary*, 1967). Although a great deal of progress has been made in the past decade regarding the nature and treatment particularly of adult stuttering, we do not yet, nor may we ever, have the luxury of being complacent with a single approach to stuttering. The variations among stutterers are too great to encompass all stutterers in one framework. Undoubtedly there are subgroups of stutterers, whose members can be grouped according to similarities in the psychosocial, physiological, and psycholinguistic makeups of the individuals. We examine these factors in detail, along with their diagnostic and therapeutic implications, later in the book.

A word of caution is warranted regarding eclecticism. An eclectic approach should be based on a well-reasoned set of principles derived from sound theoretical bases and empirical research. Eclecticism is governed by rationale and is arrived at only after an examination of the stutterer's particular symptomatology and a thorough search for a match of "best fit" between symptoms and treatment. Eclecticism is not a potpourri of therapy techniques thrown together without a priori reasoning.

DEFINITION OF FLUENCY,
NONFLUENCY, AND STUTTERING/DISFLUENCY

Stuttering has most often been defined as a disorder of fluency. The normal flow of speech is disrupted so that the timing and rhythm of speech are improperly patterned. Stuttering is defined in terms of a set of acoustic as well as visual cues. Stuttering is also defined in terms of the speaker's and listener's reaction to such cues. Because the criteria for stuttering consist of objective and subjective attributes, the task of distinguishing normal from abnormal fluency can be elusive, particularly during early childhood.

The problem is further compounded because even normal speakers show some degree of fluency disruption. Occasional fragmentations in the flow of speech and language, for example, appear in the speech of most preschoolers at one time or another during the formative years of development. Yairi (1981) found that the occasional fluency breaks observed in normal 2-year-olds not only showed great individual diversity such that "group averages lose much of their practical meaning" (p. 495), but also that the fluency breaks of 2-year-olds "already contain every single category, including sound prolongation and tense pause, which has been identified by past investigators in speech of older speakers" (p. 494).

The sections that follow define the terminology that is used throughout the book.

Fluency

"Fluency" refers to the general phenomenon of the flow or rate of speech. Overall rate pattern is influenced by the duration of individual sounds and syllables, the duration of sounds and syllables in relation to adjacent sounds and syllables, the duration of pauses, the presence of stress contrasts, and the degree of coarticulation (Starkweather, 1980). Perception of the appropriateness of fluency is affected not only by objective measures such as those just mentioned, but also by the listener's judgment of the appropriateness of these measures in terms of the thought unit and the linguistic unit of the utterance. For example, pauses should coincide with the end of a linguistic clause or sentence. The perception of excessive or inappropriate use of fillers (e.g., *um* and *uh*) and part-word repetitions (e.g., "I thi-, thi-, think it is the right place.") leads to the judgment of impaired fluency.

Although "fluency" is discussed here with neutral connotations, other authors use the term to mean the opposite of disfluencies. That is, fluency connotes the continuous, forward-flowing, coordinated manner of speech (Adams, 1982). Adams is quick to point out, however, that fluency can be described more easily than it can be defined: "A definition carefully delimits and sets the boundaries of a phenomenon, and we are presently incapable of forming such precise statements regarding fluency" (p. 174).

Nonfluency

As mentioned earlier, some degree of fluency disruption accompanies normal speech and language development. Characteristics that differentiate normal from pathological fluency are discussed later. Using Dalton and Hardcastle's (1976) terminology, "nonfluency" refers to the disruptions in the timing and flow of speech, such as interjections or phrase repetitions, that are often perceived as being part of the normal interruptions of speech. "Disfluency" refers to a breakdown in fluency that is perceived to be abnormal.

Stuttering/Disfluency

According to Van Riper (1982), "Stuttering occurs when the forward flow of speech is interrupted by a motorically disrupted sound, syllable, or word, or by the speaker's reaction thereto" (p. 15). Speech is a highly complex, patterned, and coordinated phenomenon. Although speech-language pathology students most often think of characteristics such as syllable repetition and phonatory blockage when discussing stuttering, disfluencies are also affected by variables such as rate, pitch, loudness, inflections, and articulation, as well as certain nonvocal characteristics including facial expression and postural adjustments of the speaker (Bloodstein, 1981). Adams (1982) characterizes the effects of disfluencies on speech with the descriptors "delay, interrupt, effortful, discoordination."

It is difficult to capture the complexity of stuttering in a concise definition. Nonetheless, the essence of a definition of stuttering consists of anomalies in the flow or rate of speech that are minimally distinguished by involuntary (Wingate, 1964) repetitions and prolongations, particularly of units of utterances smaller than a word. Wingate (1976) refers to the audible and silent repetitions and prolongations as the "universal and distinctive features" of stuttering.

A THREE-FACTOR MODEL FOR THE ASSESSMENT AND TREATMENT OF CHILDHOOD STUTTERING

Stuttering results from a lack of synergism or coordination between several major factors. Reflecting our broadly based and eclectic view of childhood stuttering, and to organize information about the topic, we propose a model (Myers and Wall, 1982) consisting of three interlocking circles as

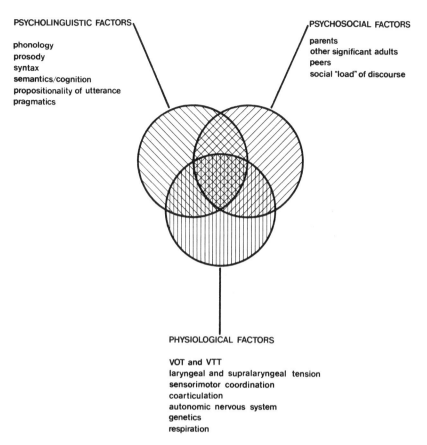

PSYCHOLINGUISTIC FACTORS

phonology
prosody
syntax
semantics/cognition
propositionality of utterance
pragmatics

PSYCHOSOCIAL FACTORS

parents
other significant adults
peers
social "load" of discourse

PHYSIOLOGICAL FACTORS

VOT and VTT
laryngeal and supralaryngeal tension
sensorimotor coordination
coarticulation
autonomic nervous system
genetics
respiration

Figure 1. Factors influencing early childhood stuttering. Reprinted by permission of the publisher from "Toward an integrated approach to early childhood stuttering," by Myers & Wall in Journal of Fluency Disorders, Vol. 7, p. 49. Copyright 1982 by Elsevier Science Publishing Co., Inc.

shown in Figure 1. The model, serving as a framework for the book, represents three factors and their respective variables, which are pertinent to the clinical management of childhood stuttering. These three factors consist of the psychosocial, physiological, and psycholinguistic characteristics and possible etiological variables of stuttering. The intersection of any two of the factors indicates the influence of one factor on another, or the likelihood that one variable, such as environmental stress, may be subsumed under two or more factors (e.g., the psychosocial and physiological factors). The physiological and psycholinguistic factors are dealt with in separate chapters. The all-pervasive psychosocial factor, however, is discussed in Chapters 3, 6, and 8. For convenience, the theories of stuttering and their therapeutic implications are discussed in terms of the three factors.

REFERENCES

Adams, M. 1982. Fluency, nonfluency, and stuttering in children. J. Fluency Disord. 7:171–185.

Bloodstein, O. 1981. A Handbook on Stuttering. 3rd Ed. National Easter Seal Society for Crippled Children and Adults, Chicago.

Dalton, P., and Hardcastle, W. 1976. Disorders of Fluency and Their Effects on Communication. Elsevier North-Holland, New York.

Johnson, W. 1939. Language and speech hygiene. General Semantic Monographs. Institute of General Semantics, Chicago.

Myers, F., and Wall, M. 1982. Toward an integrated approach to early childhood stuttering. J. Fluency Disord. 7:47–54.

Starkweather, C. 1980. Speech fluency and its development in normal children. In: N. Lass (ed.), Speech and Language: Advances in Basic Research and Practice, pp. 143–200, Vol. 4. Academic Press, New York.

Van Riper, C. 1973. The Treatment of Stuttering. Prentice-Hall, Englewood Cliffs, N.J.

Van Riper, C. 1982. The Nature of Stuttering. 2nd Ed. Prentice-Hall, Englewood Cliffs, N.J.

Wingate, M. 1964. A standard definition of stuttering. J. Speech Hear. Disord. 29:484–489.

Wingate, M. 1976. Stuttering: Theory and Treatment. John Wiley & Sons, New York.

Yairi, E. 1981. Disfluencies of normally speaking two-year-old children. J. Speech Hear. Res. 24:490–495.

2
Theories of Stuttering and Therapeutic Implications

For the student of speech and language pathology, the study of stuttering may be a confusing, even overwhelming experience—decades of research must be evaluated to find support, or lack thereof, for the various proposed theoretical frameworks. The research is voluminous and frequently contradictory. This chapter does not attempt to appraise the bulk of the research pertaining to theoretical issues of stuttering because two recent publications admirably perform this function (Bloodstein, 1981; Van Riper, 1982). Rather, it addresses the main issues of the theories and discusses their relevance to clinical practice. In addition to the publications cited above, the reader's attention is drawn to the following excellent reviews of research that relate to theory: Andrews et al. (1983), "Stuttering: A Review of Research Findings and Theories circa 1982," St. Louis (1979), "Linguistic and Motor Aspects of Stuttering," and Starkweather (1982a), "Stuttering and Laryngeal Behavior: A Review."

As professionals we are accustomed to seeking theoretical knowledge as a sound basis for clinical practice and techniques. The theoretical bases of stuttering therapy have not been on very firm ground because there is no existing theory that satisfactorily explains stuttering. The therapy that we propose is based in part on practices found to be effective, in part on our knowledge of beginning stuttering, and in part on findings in areas such as psycholinguistics and the physiology of speech. Therapy for the stutterer may be empirically based, theoretically based, or some of both. "Therapy cannot await a comprehensive, consistent theory" (Wingate, 1976). Nevertheless, the continuing growth of scientific knowledge permits evaluation of the strengths and weaknesses of existing theories; and weaker theories, such as psychodynamic theory, are recognized as having less explanatory power for stuttering than was once thought. Genetic theory, on the other hand, has acquired considerable respectability in light of recent scientific research.

This discussion of theories of stuttering and their therapeutic implications is organized according to the psychosocial factor, the physiological factor, and the psycholinguistic factor, assuming some interaction among the three factors. Within this framework, however, we refer to theories attempting to explain the etiology of stuttering, the maintenance and development of stuttering, and what Bloodstein (1981) calls "the moment of stuttering."

THE PSYCHOSOCIAL FACTOR

Psychodynamic Theory

Under "psychodynamic theory" we consider problems of adjustment of individuals as well as more severe disorders usually associated with psychoanalytic thinking. The "lay" perception of stuttering as an emotional disorder is very strong. Invite a fairly naive speech pathology class to contribute information on "the cause" of stuttering and the responses probably will be evenly divided among "psychological problems," "emotional problems," and "nervousness," with perhaps some mention of parental demands and high expectations of the young child learning to speak. Some of these observations have been verified in data collected by Cooper (1975, 1979) and St. Louis and Lass (1981) with speech pathology students and clinicians as subjects. Cooper designed the Clinical Attitudes Toward Stuttering (CATS) Inventory and sent it to 142 school clinicians in two states; St. Louis and Lass (1981) analyzed CATS questionnaires from 1,902 speech pathology students (freshman to doctoral) from 33 states. Examples of responses are as follows. To the statement "Most stutterers have psychological problems," 50% of Cooper's and 54% of St. Louis and Lass's subjects agreed; to the statement "Most stutterers possess feelings of inferiority," 58% of Cooper's and 71% of St. Louis and Lass's agreed; to the statement "Some personality traits are characteristic of stutterers," 49% of Cooper's and 54% of St. Louis and Lass's subjects agreed.

Cooper pointed out that clinicians have maintained erroneous impressions of stutterers, despite evidence to the contrary. That is, the evidence suggests that stutterers do not possess characteristic personality traits, and typically they do not have personality disorders. Since the genetic and physiological aspects of stuttering have assumed considerable importance in recent years, it is a little surprising that many clinicians cling to a psychodynamic frame of reference for stuttering.

Psychodynamic theory in a psychoanalytic framework was originally based on Freud's view of personality and psychosocial development. Since Freud stressed the importance of an "oral" stage and an "anal" stage in the child's maturation, some psychoanalysts structured a theory of stuttering around those stages. Coriat (1927, 1931, 1943), for example, regarded stuttering as the result of an oral fixation. Fenichel (1945) and Heilpern (1941) opted for a fixation at the anal stage of development. Glauber (1958), however, believed that the stutterer suffered from a conflict between the id and the superego. Travis (1971) presented the "unspeakable feelings" of stutterers as the reason for their ambivalence about speaking, and Barbara (1954, 1965) suggested that inadequate interpersonal relationships and adjustment to life situations affect the speech of the stutterer.

Researchers have explored results of projective tests such as the Rorschach and "personality tests" such as the Minnesota Multiphasic Personality Inventory (MMPI) on adults, and, where applicable, on children. Their interest was in finding out whether stutterers differ from nonstutterers in personality or in psychological makeup. Van Riper, having summarized this research, commented as follows:

> *Despite the fact that we have scrutinized all of these investigations*
> *with some care, it is difficult to fit them together into a coherent*
> *judgment. So many of them fail to fulfill basic criteria of good*
> *research. So many of them contradict each other. The case for*
> *stuttering as a neurosis and only a neurosis has not been made*
> (Van Riper, 1982, p. 272).

Andrews et al. (1983) pointed out that if differences between stutterers and nonstutterers are to be viewed as causative agents, the differences must be present before or when the child begins to stutter. Later differences may represent factors that inhibit remission or factors that result from stuttering. These investigators noted that stutterers, on the whole, show more difficulties with social adjustment than nonstutterers, but that this is probably a consequence rather than a cause of stuttering.

All things considered, psychological maladjustment has not been established as a cause for stuttering. Some stutterers react to their stuttering, and some listeners react to stutterers. It is possible, therefore, to have emotionality surrounding stuttering without it being a causative agent. Also, it has not been established that emotionality does surround stuttering in all cases.

Therapeutic Implications   A treatment for stuttering derived from psychodynamic theory would by implication use psychoanalysis or some form of psychotherapy. The failure of this type of therapy to deal effectively with stuttering, however, militates against the therapy and the theory (Van Riper, 1958, 1971, 1982; Webster, 1977). There has been no satisfactory documentation of psychoanalysis or psychotherapy as the effective treatment method for stutterers. Reports that an occasional stutterer has improved with this method of treatment, or any other method, should not beguile the beginning clinician into thinking that it is, therefore, the preferred method of treatment for all or most stutterers.

If we apply the theoretical framework to the treatment of children, some type of play therapy in which the child acts out his feelings and interactions with those in the environment, in the presence of a benevolent and informed adult clinician, would be indicated. In the 1950's when psychoanalytic theory enjoyed greater popularity, such therapy with young children was practiced. The implication was that many stutterers were troubled children. The current trend toward techniques dealing more directly with youngsters' speech, and toward more language-oriented therapies, reflects a change of focus.

It is possible, of course, for a stutterer of any age to be extremely troubled about speech, or troubled for other reasons. Some form of psychological help may then be necessary, but based on current information, it is not the preferred method of treatment for all stutterers. This point of view with regard to adults was confirmed by Van Riper (1958), who systematically documented the results of therapies he used on adult stutterers, and then carried out extensive followup evaluations. He found that psychotherapy alone gave very poor results.

Summary   No hard evidence is available to support a psychodynamic theory of stuttering. The mild adjustment problems exhibited by some stutterers seem to result from stuttering, not to cause it. In addition, psychotherapy and psychoanalysis have generally not been effective in remediating stuttering. The need for such therapy, as an adjunct to stuttering therapy or in lieu of it, should be decided on an individual basis.

Diagnosogenic Theory

Wendell Johnson believed that children become stutterers only after being "diagnosed" as stutterers by those in their immediate environment, usually one or both parents (Johnson, 1955; Johnson and Associates, 1959). According to Johnson, the diagnosed children experienced routine nonfluencies of early childhood until the time of the diagnosis, but the attention drawn to their speech production by anxious parents with perfectionistic attitudes about speech and child raising resulted in the automatic act of speech becoming a highly conscious act. The children's increased awareness of the manner of speech production led to increased tension and an "anticipatory avoidance reaction," thus beginning the cycle of increased tension and increased force of speech in an effort to avoid speech difficulties. The end result was blocking, further anticipation, and tension. According to Bloodstein, the basic tenet of the diagnosogenic theory is that ". . . at the moment of initial diagnosis the speech of children who come to be regarded as stutterers does not differ in essential respects from that of children who do not come to be so regarded" (Bloodstein, 1981, p. 297).

As supportive data for his hypothesis, Johnson used results from his large scale study that compared the onset of nonfluencies, as recalled by the parents, of the young stutterers with that of young nonstutterers (Johnson and Associates, 1959). In evaluating his data, Johnson stressed the overlap of the categories in the two groups of children. Except for "complete block," which seldom occurred even in the experimental group, some of each type of disfluency occurred in both stutterers and nonstutterers. Johnson hypothesized, therefore, that some parents perceived a characteristic as stuttering and others did not. See Chapter 7 for further discussion of this theory.

In a subsequent refinement of the theory, Johnson proposed the "interaction hypothesis" containing a three-part interaction: the interaction of the listener (who presumably is sensitive to the speaker's disfluency), the degree of disfluency of the speaker, and the speaker's sensitivity to his or her disfluency and to the evaluative reactions of others.

Johnson's theories infer specific reactions of significant adults to the child, namely, reactions of anxiety and perfectionism, because the adults react to something in their children that other parents take for granted or ignore. Research has not demonstrated, however, that the parents of stutterers, as a group, possess such reactions; nor has research demonstrated that the parents of stutterers are, as a group, more neurotic than the parents of nonstutterers (Andrews et al., 1983). Johnson apparently rejected the possibility that the fluency of some young children is disrupted to such an extent that it warrants parental attention. Parental concern is appropriate, however, if repetitions and prolongations are present to an unusual degree in a child's speech. A number of factors, including environmental, then may determine the course of the disruptions—whether they subside, get worse, subside and return, remain stable—there are several possibilities.

In previously mentioned studies by Cooper (1975, 1979) and St. Louis and Lass (1981) in which school clinicians and speech pathology students reacted to various statements pertaining to the emotional well-being of stutterers, approximately 25% of the clinicians and students polled indicated that they consider parents to be the causative agents of stuttering. This is a high figure in view of the paucity of supporting data. On the other hand, the genetic studies discussed in this chapter suggest that environmental influences must be involved in the onset of some cases of stuttering. Although the nature of that involvement is still obscure, there is a growing interest in examining the nuances of the verbal interaction between parent and child. A single-subject study by Guitar et al. (1981), for example, examined pragmatic aspects of discourse between a young stutterer and a parent, in an attempt to discover possible relationships between stuttering and such pragmatics (see "Dealing with Pragmatics," in Chapter 8). This work is in its early stages and there are no conclusions to be drawn, but we await further developments with interest.

Therapeutic Implications   Johnson's diagnosogenic theory implies a therapy for the beginning stutterer that is indirect, and is aimed at changing perfectionistic attitudes in the parents of the child through counseling. Chapter 7 summarizes Johnson's orientation to therapy.

Johnson developed a method based on the anticipatory avoidance concept for treating older and more advanced stutterers. That is, he considered the stutterer's difficulties with speech to be efforts to avoid stuttering. Johnson's therapy proposes a semantic reorientation to the stutterer, one in which there is considerable reevaluation of the self, of what the stutterer does with the lips, or with respiration, for example, to prevent speech from emerging. The client is to think of what he or she is doing to prevent smooth speech production from occurring, rather than thinking that the stuttering is doing something to the client. This semantic alteration is combined with other aspects of therapy, such as evaluating the nonfluencies of nonstutterers, to foster awareness that fluency and nonfluency are something of a continuum rather than dichotomous events for the stutterer and nonstutterer.

Summary   The diagnosogenic theory was the first well-reasoned theory offered to explain the onset of stuttering. The interaction hypothesis, which followed as a refinement of the theory, was in fact more subtle and thorough, but it did not gain the popularity that its predecessor achieved. Johnson's thinking had a profound and far-reaching effect on therapeutic considerations of stuttering, particularly with young children. His idea that early stuttering is influenced by pressures from parents and other environmental sources is still accepted. The extent to which the pressures may "cause" stuttering, however, as Johnson claimed, is unknown, although it seems logical that they may act to maintain or exacerbate existing stuttering in the child. Attempts to delineate the pressure, as in studies of parental anxiety, have been inconclusive, but more focused studies on the kinds of verbal interaction that take place between parent and child may offer insight into environmental influences.

The Anticipatory Struggle Hypothesis

The anticipatory struggle hypothesis is an account of "the moment of stuttering" rather than a theory of etiology (Bloodstein, 1972, 1981). It seeks to explain the occurrence of the stuttering block by suggesting that stutterers interfere with speech production because they believe that speech is inherently difficult. That is, stutterers stutter because they perceive speech as requiring special attention and effort. This perception may be based in the reality of a disorder such as cluttering, language delay, or articulation disorder and/or, social (mis)evaluations of speech. Whatever the reason for the perceived difficulty, the stutterers' efforts to avoid it constitute the symptoms of stuttering. Bloodstein places the anticipatory struggle hypothesis in a historical perspective, with its roots partially, for example, in Wendell Johnson's anticipatory avoidance reaction.

With regard to the onset of stuttering, Bloodstein has proposed the "continuity hypothesis," which incorporates his long-held concern about young stutterers' language and speech skills as related to their disfluencies (Bloodstein, 1958, 1975, 1981). Rather than approach the onset of stuttering as a misdiagnosis of normal nonfluencies, as Johnson did, Bloodstein suggested that the child might develop reactions to speech production either because of external stress, or, as stated earlier, because of a belief that speech is difficult. The external stress might be parental criticism of the child's speech, perhaps resulting from unrealistically high standards or parental ignorance about language and speech acquisition. Bloodstein's terms "tension" and "fragmentation" describe the resulting effects on speech production when the child anticipates failure in speaking, whatever the reason. Anticipatory struggle develops in the child's efforts to produce speech well. Tension may result in hard attacks on stop consonants and prolongation of continuants. Speech may become fragmented at a word level, as in *mo-mo-mommy,* or at a syntactic level where the repetition would occur at the onset of a phrase or clause.

The continuity aspect of the hypothesis lies in Bloodstein's belief that the stuttering of the young child has its origins in the nonfluencies of normal speech and language acquisition, and that the young stutterer's symptoms are an "extreme degree" of normal nonfluencies.

Outlining his hypothesis of the etiology of stuttering, Bloodstein states:

> *Stuttering is an anticipatory struggle reaction. In its clinical form it represents a relatively severe degree of tensions and fragmentations that are a common occurrence in the speech of normal young children. It develops readily in circumstances in which speech pressures are unusually heavy, the child's vulnerability to them unusually high, or the provocations in the form of communicative difficulties or failures unusually frequent, severe, or chronic* (Bloodstein, 1981, p. 336).

Therapeutic Implications　　The continuity hypothesis suggests that at least for young stutterers, therapy should aim at increasing the clients' sense of confidence about speech and about themselves as speakers. This may involve fairly conventional counseling on handling fluent and disfluent days, reinforcing fluency, and dealing with any "demanding, restrictive or perfectionistic" tendencies in the parents.

Such techniques should prevent or reduce the children's anticipation of difficulty. Presumably they then struggle less, physical tension subsides, anticipation lessens, and speech becomes easier.

Assisting the older, confirmed stutterer in dealing with anticipatory struggle implies using methods that will in time reduce the expectation of stuttering and the struggle associated with speech. To reduce the expectation of stuttering and the stutterer's struggle, indirect methods such as Johnson's semantic reorientation in addition to more direct techniques, such as those used in Frick's (1970) motor planning (see Chapter 7), seem to be appropriate. An "unlearning" process in therapy is implied by this theory. Therapy needs to help the stutterer to unlearn the belief that speech is difficult, and to unlearn that one must try hard and struggle to talk.

Summary   The anticipatory struggle hypothesis proposes that the stutterer's speech becomes increasingly fragmented because of his or her perception that speech is, in some way, difficult, and anticipatory struggle results. This hypothesis may be viewed as an explanation of the moment of stuttering. Bloodstein, however, also incorporates anticipatory struggle into his explanation of the etiology of stuttering—the continuity hypothesis. The continuity hypothesis proposes that stuttering emanates from normal tensions and fragmentations of speech in young children. The child, under pressure, may develop anticipation of speech difficulty and anticipatory struggle, with the resulting increase in tensions and fragmentations of speech. The continuity hypothesis suggests that there is no sharp distinction between the speech pattern of young stutterers and nonstutterers.

Learning Theory

Learning theory, first developed in the field of psychology, has stimulated the formation of theories of the etiology, the development, and the moment of stuttering. The two-factor theory, the theory of operant conditioning, and the approach-avoidance conflict theory are representative of these points of view.

Brutten and Shoemaker's (1967) two-factor theory incorporates both classical and instrumental (or operant) conditioning. These investigators use classical conditioning to explain the onset of stuttering and speech-related anxiety, and instrumental conditioning to explain the development of associated (secondary, accessory) symptoms. In essence, they consider that the child's stuttering results from negative emotional arousal that is triggered by stressful environmental events. The authors note that speech disruptions can occur under conditions of emotional (or autonomic nervous system) stress or arousal, and that these disruptions co-occur with the negative emotions. The negative emotions—with attendant speech breakdown—may be conditioned by the recurrence of, and pairing with, the stressful environmental events or cues. Classical conditioning is denoted by the pairing of the conditioned stimulus (environmental stress) with the unconditioned stimulus (negative emotions). In time, the disfluent responses may generalize to other similar situations. Then the child is thought to begin to exert effort over speech attempts to control them; perhaps tightening the articulators, or stamping the foot to get the word out, thus beginning the use of associated features that worsen the condition. According to Brutten and Shoemaker, these associated symptoms are "adjustive" or "problem-solving" behaviors. Insofar as these behaviors might be intermittently effective or "rewarding" to the stutterers—because they provide temporary relief—they reinforce the condition. The learning of the associated symptoms is strengthened by the variability of their effectiveness; that is, they do not always "work" for the stutterer, but sometimes they do. This means that the stutterer is intermittently reinforced for their use, and through avoidance learning, they become part of the symptomatology. For further information on avoidance learning and stuttering see Van Riper (1971, 1982) and Starkweather (1982b).

In contrast to Brutten and Shoemaker's two-factor theory, Shames and Sherrick (1963) propose that stuttering results from operant conditioning alone. They suggest that the child's normal nonfluencies might be reinforced by, for example, parental attention. As a result, there could be an increase in nonfluencies, which might then be punished, resulting in alteration of the nonfluencies to struggle and silence. The newer stuttering pattern is negatively reinforced by termination of the punishment but in time will probably incur further punishment. Thus, the repetitions and prolongations deteriorate into a pattern that is learned and strengthened through fluctuating schedules of reinforcement. In addition to the negative reinforcement of stuttering, there may also be positive reinforcement, because the child may get more attention from his listeners when exhibiting disfluencies. Shames and Sherrick regard any kind of nonfluency as an operant that can be increased or decreased by some type of reinforcement.

Shames and Sherrick's point of view is not universally accepted, partly because the evidence from behavior modification studies—that operant procedures predictably influence stuttering—is not entirely clearcut (see Van Riper, 1982, for a review of such studies). In addition, despite the large body of operant research pertaining to stuttering, its relation to the etiology of stuttering remains unclear.

Sheehan's approach-avoidance conflict theory (1953, 1958) hypothesized that the stutterer becomes caught between two drives: the drive to talk in order to communicate, and the drive not to talk. If the drive to talk is stronger than the drive not to talk, Sheehan reasoned, the speaker will go ahead and will experience fluency. If the avoidance drive is stronger, the individual will remain silent. Stuttering occurs when the two drives are of equal strength, and the speaker oscillates between them. The going ahead and pulling back are manifested as stuttering and represent a theory of the moment of stuttering.

Furthermore, Sheehan posited that if the stutterer fails to go ahead and talk, he suffers the consequences of frustration and guilt. If he succeeds in going ahead, he suffers the shame and guilt that accompany the stuttering, thus creating a double approach-avoidance conflict.

An interesting aspect of Sheehan's theory is his application of it to different levels of the stutterer's life. That is, the conflict may occur on a word level, a situational level, a level of emotional expression, or a level of interpersonal relationships. Given our current knowledge, however, it seems unlikely that most stutterers possess the multiple conflicts that

Sheehan suggests or that they would experience them for each moment of stuttering.

Therapeutic Implications   Classical conditioning may involve arousal of the autonomic nervous system with its attendant emotional discomfort; therefore desensitization procedures, which are designed to systematically reduce the emotional state of the client in specific situations, are implemented. For operant or instrumental conditioning, where learning depends on the reinforcement of a particular behavior, the therapeutic approach is usually to reinforce fluency, to punish stuttering, or to modify the stuttering.

Brutten and Shoemaker (1967) formulated a therapy to dovetail with their two-factor theory of the etiology and maintenance of stuttering. It incorporates deep muscle relaxation and systematic desensitization of the classically conditioned reactions such as anxiety (adapted from Wolpe, 1958). When the client is relaxed, he or she imagines feared speaking situations in a hierarchical fashion, from least feared to most feared, continuing up the hierarchy until each imagined situation can be tolerated without a fearful reaction. The associated symptoms are treated by massed practice (i.e., the voluntary, repeated production of a behavior (response) in the absence of reinforcement to achieve extinction of that behavior), designed to result in reactive inhibition of the symptoms.

Operant conditioning is commonly used to ameliorate or to assist in the amelioration of stuttering, regardless of whether the clinician assumes that it has a role in the etiology and/or the maintenance and development of the condition. The behavior modification studies that began in the 1950's instigated a variety of treatment techniques for stuttering therapy. The techniques included punishment to decrease the stuttering, such as electric shock (e.g., Daly and Cooper, 1967; Daly and Frick, 1970), and time-out (e.g., Costello, 1975, 1980; Haroldson, Martin, and Starr, 1968; Martin and Haroldson, 1971). In addition, time-out (Costello, 1975; Martin, Kuhl, and Anderson, 1972) and verbal punishment (Reed and Godden, 1977) have been tried on a limited number of young children.

Another technique related to learning theory and behavior modification is the withdrawal of the proposed positive reinforcer of stuttering in children—namely, parental attention. This is exemplified by L. J. Johnson's (1980) work with young stutterers, whose parents were advised not to respond to the stuttered speech (see Chapter 7).

A powerful influence of behavior modification may be seen in the fluency shaping techniques now being used for the treatment of stutterers. Such techniques reinforce the stutterer's fluent speech. They have been frequently incorporated into "programs" that use operant principles in a highly organized fashion, and specify the type of reinforcement to be used, schedules of reinforcement, and series of steps designed to lead the stutterer, ideally, to fluent speech (Ryan, 1974, 1979; Ryan and Van Kirk, 1974; Webster, 1974, 1979).

Sheehan's conceptualization of stuttering, needless to say, does not lend itself to the techniques just described. The implication from his theory is that the approach drive must be strengthened and the avoidance drive reduced. The various "levels" of Sheehan's theory may be therapeutically sensible for some stutterers, who may be helped by recognizing and learning to cope with ambivalence about, for example, speaking feared words and speaking in feared situations. The theory suggests a psychotherapeutic approach to stuttering therapy, which may incorporate techniques to modify the blocking.

Summary   The examples of learning theory presented attempt to account for the onset of stuttering through classical conditioning—Brutten and Shoemaker, and through operant (instrumental) conditioning—Shames and Sherrick. They attempt to account for the maintenance and development of stuttering through instrumental conditioning—Brutten and Shoemaker, and to account for the moment of stuttering through the approach-avoidance conflict theory—Sheehan. Learning theory seems to have more explanatory power for the maintenance and development of stuttering than for the onset or the moment of stuttering. Behavior modification techniques, an offshoot of learning theory, have become widely used in stuttering therapy.

Highlights of the Psychosocial Factor

Psychodynamic theory, the diagnosogenic theory, the anticipatory struggle hypothesis, and the continuity hypothesis, together with learning theory, all constitute the psychosocial factor. The diagnosogenic theory has substantially influenced thinking on the cause and treatment of stuttering, but its power has recently subsided with the advent of newer information. The anticipatory struggle hypothesis and the continuity hypothesis have some sound therapeutic implications, regardless of whether one accepts the tenet basic to the continuity hypothesis—that stuttering emanates from normal nonfluency. Learning theory has contributed more to our understanding of the maintenance and development of stuttering than to our knowledge of etiology. It also underlies the organization of stuttering modification and fluency-shaping techniques used in many therapies.

Psychosocial factors are difficult to delineate and to measure. Their relative impact on a child in a complex environment, given that the child brings with him or her a specific set of genetic and physiological variables, is extremely difficult to gauge. Clinicians generally adhere to empirically based clinical assumptions to assist in the prevention or amelioration of stuttering, based in part on psychosocial factors. Psychodynamic theory has offered little satisfactory explanation for the onset of stuttering, and little in the way of therapy for most stutterers; psychotherapy or psycho-analysis might be relevant for selected stutterers.

THE PHYSIOLOGICAL FACTOR

References to a physiological or organic factor in stuttering apparently date back to Aristotle. For historical reviews of theories and therapies of stuttering, refer to Rieber and Wollock (1977) and Van Riper (1973). Just as neuroticism has been ruled out as the cause of stuttering within the psychosocial factor, certain anatomical and physiological phenomena seem to have been ruled out in the physiological factor, by virtue of extensive research. We are reasonably certain, for example, that neither the observable structures of the speech mechanism nor the general health of stutterers differ from that of nonstutterers. In addition, the biochemical makeup of stutterers has not been shown to differ from that of nonstut-terers. Numerous other physiological areas have been studied extensively in attempts to determine why the stutterer's speech production mechanism intermittently fails to function with the smoothness and synergism of nor-mally produced speech. For the purpose of discussion the areas have been divided into the following: the central nervous system function, peripheral speech production, and genetics.

Central Nervous System Function

Under the rubric of "central nervous system function" we consider studies of general brain function, hemispheric dominance for language and speech, reaction time, and feedback mechanisms.

General Brain Function   An unusually large number of stutterers has been reported among the Down's syndrome and retarded populations (Bloodstein, 1981). Andrews et al. (1983) suggested perinatal damage as a likely cause of stuttering, because of the high incidence of this condition in neurologically impaired populations. Some argue, however, that the symp-toms of disfluency in such populations are different from stuttering. Helm, Butler, and Canter (1980) described stuttering in a series of clients with acquired brain damage, but delineated ways in which these and other similar clients' symptoms may differ from conventional stuttering. In spite of evidence suggesting a relation between brain damage and stuttering-like symptoms, examination of stutterers' brain function by electroenceph-alography (EEG) has produced conflicting results as to whether stutterers are, on the whole, afflicted with some type of brain damage. In his extensive review of the EEG research, Van Riper (1982) concluded that a minority of stutterers exhibits brain wave abnormalities, whereas Bloodstein, reviewing the same area, draws two conclusions:

> *First, the weight of evidence from controlled, quantitative studies supports the view that, except for small differences that are difficult to account for, [stutterers'] brain potentials tend to be normal. Second, there is a considerable body of additional work that suggests the presence of brain pathology in a large proportion of stutterers, but this has not yet received sufficient confirmation from adequately controlled studies, and conflicting findings exist* (Bloodstein, 1981, pp. 128–129).

Andrews et al. (1983) regard the current body of evidence on brain potentials as equivocal and suggest more focused research on hemispheric control. Whether stutterers, or a subgroup of stutterers, have some type of brain damage, therefore, remains unclear, but there is just enough tantalizing evidence to suggest that this is a possibility.

Hemispheric Dominance for Language and Speech   Most speakers have one cerebral hemisphere dominant for language and speech production: usually, but not exclusively, the left. The question of bilateral dominance for stutterers was first raised by Samuel T. Orton (1927) and Lee Edward Travis (1931). Their theory proposed that the competing hemispheres interrupt the smooth transmission of neural impulses to the muscles responsible for speech production, causing breakdown in the stutterer's speech. Years of research into the handedness and sidedness of stutterers, however, failed to support the Orton-Travis theory of cerebral dominance. However, interest was renewed in the cerebral dominance theory with the advent of the Wada test, which consists of the injection of a solution of sodium amytal into the carotid artery. If the subject is speaking, speech is disrupted as the solution is circulated throughout the hemisphere that received the solution, provided that hemisphere is dominant for speech. Andrews et al. (1983) note that all six stutterers tested with the Wada technique had one dominant side for speech. Five stutterers with known brain damage, however, demonstrated bilateral hemispheric control. The case for bilateral cerebral dominance as evaluated by the Wada test in stutterers, therefore, has not been made.

The task of dichotic listening has also been used in attempts to establish the cerebral dominance of stutterers. Here the subject receives competing stimuli (in this case, verbal stimuli) through earphones to each ear. The task is to recall the stimuli. Subjects who report stimuli delivered to the right ear (and left hemisphere) more frequently than those delivered to the left ear (and right hemisphere) are said to have a right ear advantage (REA), which is the norm.

More studies have been carried out with the noninvasive dichotic listening procedure than with the Wada test, but these studies have given equivocal results. In examining adults, Curry and Gregory (1969), Perrin and Eisenson (1970) and Sommers, Brady, and Moore (1975), for example, found differences in ear advantage between stutterers and nonstutterers; Cerf and Prins (1974), Quinn (1972), and Rosenfield and Goodglass (1980) found no difference in ear advantage between the two groups. A small subgroup of stutterers, however, has shown a lack of clearcut dominance.

In attempting to clarify the role of cerebral dominance on stuttering in children, Cimorell-Strong, Gilbert, and Frick (1983) compared 15 stutterers and 15 nonstutterers at ages of 5, 7, and 9 years ($N = 90$). A significant difference existed between stutterers' and nonstutterers' responses to dichotic presentation. Whereas 82% of the nonstutterers exhibited a REA, only 55% of the stutterers did so. The findings suggest, as has been proposed with adult stutterers, that although children who stutter, as a group, do not exhibit incomplete laterality of speech functions, a subset of youngsters does seem to show incomplete laterality.

In smaller scale studies, Slorach and Noehr (1973) and Gruber and Powell (1974) found no difference in responses of stuttering and nonstuttering children in dichotic listening tasks.

Although the EEG studies have added little to the search for a physiological factor in stuttering, recent work of Moore and Haynes (1980), Moore and Lang (1977), and Moore and Lorendo (1980) is of interest. Examining the α-wave rhythm of the brain during linguistic tasks, Moore and his colleagues found that stutterers exhibit reduced α-wave response in the right hemisphere in comparison with nonstutterers, suggesting asymmetrical cerebral activity in stutterers. Further research is needed in this area to confirm these findings.

The search for irregularities of hemispheric dominance has been like the search for brain damage in stutterers—inconclusive but revealing possibilities. The newer work on α-wave rhythms shows promise and undoubtedly will be pursued. We anticipate further research that may help to delineate subgroups of stutterers exhibiting, for example, a lack of clearcut dominance, or reversed dominance, or normally organized hemispheric activity.

Reaction Time   Reaction time studies on stutterers have required subjects to produce a response by a muscle system (phonatory, e.g., or manual) as quickly as possible after an auditory or visual stimulus has been presented. Some consider the auditory system to be faulty in stutterers, and use of the visual system circumvents the suspect auditory system. An auditory stimulus might be a tone delivered at a specific frequency and intensity level; a visual stimulus might be a flash of light on a screen. Measurements are made of the speed with which the subject initiates the required response, such as a vowel or a syllable, upon hearing or seeing the stimulus. Additionally, the speed with which the subject ceases the response when the stimulus is withdrawn might be measured. It is generally agreed after considerable research in this area that many stutterers exhibit slower reaction times than nonstutterers in initiating phonation, whether the signal is given in the auditory or the visual mode. Also, stutterers are slower than nonstutterers in reacting with nonspeech oral or laryngeal movements, and with manual movements (see reviews by Andrews et al., 1983; Starkweather, 1982a).

The observation of the slower reaction time of the stutterer may reflect a poorly integrated central nervous system, although for laryngeal reaction times, a failure of the laryngeal musculature rather than a neural explanation has been proposed (Prosek et al., 1979). Further details of stutterers' reaction times, particularly with regard to children, are given in Chapter 5.

Feedback Mechanisms   The concept of feedback mechanisms is based on cybernetics, Norbert Wiener's (1948) term for the study of self-regulating mechanisms or servomechanisms. In such systems, errors in the output are returned to the source so that adjustments may be made within the system, and the output corrected. Speech scientists assume that because of the complexity of speech, some system of monitoring or feedback exists—even if for emergency use only (Borden, 1979)—or has existed in the developing stages of the individual's speech and language. Speech-language pathologists are clearly interested in this concept, which might lead to explanations of pathological speech production and provide avenues for remediation. Feedback, then, pertains to the capacity of a speaker to monitor speech. Such feedback may be provided through auditory channels (bone or air), through taction, proprioception, or central neural feedback (Borden, 1979; Borden and Harris, 1980).

Borden has summarized well the doubts about the necessity for ongoing feedback in the mature speaker, together with pertinent research. For example, speakers may have their auditory feedback obliterated by appropriately loud masking noise without dire consequences to speech production, although pitch and loudness levels increase somewhat. Also, speakers' taction may be disturbed through nerve block injections that interfere with branches of the trigeminal nerve. Again, only minor disruptions of speech production occur. Proprioception may be impaired experimentally by mechanical interference with normal proprioception, and again through nerve blocks presumed to affect the proprioceptive system. In the case of mechanical interference with the customary placement of the articulators, subjects compensated for the interference. In attempts to block neural proprioception, there has been no perceptible interference with speech production.

Finally, a method of central internal feedback has been proposed based on knowledge of the central nervous system (CNS). It suggests that motor impulses are monitored in the CNS as soon as they leave the cerebral cortex. This means that on the basis of previously stored patterns, the system can correct itself before neural impulses reach the peripheral level (Borden, 1979; Borden and Harris, 1980). This is a sophisticated and plausible theoretical construct that has not, of course, lent itself to verification.

Van Riper (1982) proposes that a child may begin to acquire spoken language using auditory feedback to match output against the model of others. Then, a gradual shift may occur from auditory to proprioceptive feedback, so that audition is freed for other purposes. Because the two systems may function more or less simultaneously for awhile, interference between the auditory and proprioceptive signals may cause broken words. When proprioception assumes the job of monitoring the speech-motor sequences, the overload is reduced. According to Van Riper's model, the normally speaking adult is thought to monitor his or her speech "somasthetically."

Interest in the feedback system of stutterers has prompted investigation of the effects on rate of stuttering when feedback systems are disrupted. This work has focused on the more accessible systems—auditory and tactile. When masking noise is delivered to the stutterer at high intensity levels, stuttering rate is reduced (see, e.g., Adams and Moore, 1972; Cherry and Sayers, 1956; Conture, 1974; Maraist and Hutton, 1957; Shane, 1955). Some researchers maintain that stuttering is reduced because the noise cuts out any aberrant functioning of the auditory system, such as an abnormal acoustic reflex (Webster, 1974; Webster and Dorman, 1971) or abnormal auditory feedback (Stromsta, 1956, 1959, 1972). The case for an abnormal acoustic reflex, however, has not been established (see Hannley and Dorman (1982) for a review of this research), and efforts to prove that the stutterer has some type of delayed auditory feedback have also been unsuccessful (see reviews by Bloodstein, 1981; Van Riper, 1982; Wingate, 1976). Wingate explains the masking effect by citing the tendency of speakers in noise to raise their vocal intensity (the Lombard effect), suggesting that the change in phonation somehow effects the change in rate of stuttering.

As contrasted to masking noise, delayed auditory feedback (DAF) refers to the postponement in auditory feedback of speech when a speaker's utterance is fed back through earphones a fraction of a second after it was spoken. Lee (1950, 1951) discovered that such a delay tends to disrupt a normal speaker's fluency. He called this phenomenon "artificial stuttering," inferring a similarity between normal speech under DAF conditions, and stuttering. His work led to speculation that the auditory feedback system of the stutterer might be disrupted, and that this in some way resulted in a speech breakdown similar to that of a normal speaker's breakdown under conditions of artificial delay. There has been argument over whether a normal speaker's production under DAF and a stutterer's speech pattern are dissimilar (Neelley, 1961) or similar (Yates, 1963), and therefore whether the question of an intrinsic delay for the stutterer is plausible. However, as stated previously, the case for distorted auditory feedback as a cause of stuttering has not been made.

DAF research with children has sought to clarify the role of auditory feedback on young fluent speakers, and to a lesser extent, on young stutterers. Several investigators (e.g., Chase et al., 1961; Cullen et al., 1968; Yeni-Komshian, Chase, and Mobley, 1968) suggested that DAF is a more potent disrupter to children's fluency as age increases. This research used a delay of 200 msec, and more disruption to children's speech was found with an increase in age. Such findings argue against the notion that young children rely heavily on auditory feedback and argue against Van Riper's proposal that stuttering may begin when feedback for speech shifts from the important auditory channel to the proprioceptive. Studies using variable time delays, however, reported more reliance on auditory feedback in young children. Both Mackay (1968) and Siegel et al. (1980) found that DAF disrupted the speech of 5-year-olds more than that of 8-year-olds, and of the 8-year-olds more than that of adults. Furthermore, the longer the delay for the children, the more the disruption—particularly for the 5-year-olds. The more detailed studies, therefore, seem to demonstrate that auditory feedback is important to younger speakers and that they depend on it less with maturation.

Although an interesting phenomenon, DAF has failed to clarify theoretical issues of stuttering and has not added to our knowledge of its etiology. As indicated under "Clinical Implications," however, it has added to our repertoire of clinical techniques, because generally speaking severe adult stutterers reduce disfluencies when speaking under DAF (Bloodstein, 1981; Van Riper, 1982). It appears to have been used little clinically with children; limited use is reported in the clinical section later in this chapter. Timmons and Boudreau (1978) examined the speech of 25 stutterers and nonstutterers, average age 9 years, using variable time delays. The groups behaved similarly, in that they were more disfluent at the longer delay times and more fluent at the shorter delay times. There was no difference in speaking times and no difference in the number of disfluencies between the groups at the various delay times. Further exploration of the effects of DAF on children may lead to increased clinical use of the technique on this population, although not with very young children, who might be frightened by the procedure (see Adams, 1980).

The focus of the feedback research on stuttering has been on the auditory channel rather than taction and proprioception. Hutchinson and Ringel (1975), however, studied the speech of six stutterers whose oral areas were anesthetized; they found an increase in the rate and severity of stuttering, with prolongation particularly affected. Hutchinson and Ringel's results suggest that the stutterers may have been quite dependent on feedback from the peripheral speech mechanism for the organization of speech. The results may suggest, as the authors proposed, that as a result of the loss of sensory feedback, the stutterers were unable to reduce the blocks by compensatory oral gestures. Or, the increased rate of stuttering may be due to infiltration by the anesthesia of the motor system for speech production (Borden, 1979), thereby further disrupting the stutterers' attempts at speech production.

To summarize the CNS influences on stuttering, stutterers, on the whole, do not exhibit detectable brain damage or confusion of cerebral dominance. However, the possibility of a subgroup of stutterers possessing one or other of these conditions has not been ruled out. Reaction time studies have almost consistently demonstrated differences in performance between stutterers and nonstutterers. If one subscribes to the tenet that reaction time reflects the integrity of the CNS, then certainly there is evidence of a lack in the stutterers, but the reaction time differences may reflect peripheral events. Feedback mechanisms have been explored fairly extensively in the auditory mode, and sparsely in the tactile and proprioceptive modes. There are no data to suggest that the stutterer's auditory mechanism or auditory feedback are different from those of nonstutterers. With regard to tactile and proprioceptive feedback, there are too few data to permit a judgment.

Therapeutic Implications   The suspicion persists that some kind of asymmetry of the cerebral hemispheres or some slight aberration of the CNS may have a subtle effect on the timing of the physiology of the stutterer's speech. The "handedness" aspect of cerebral dominance, however, has not been established. That is, changing a child's handedness is generally not considered to lead to stuttering and is not considered to be a cure for stuttering.

More recent thinking on the physiology of stuttering has led to some increased support for a symptomatic approach to therapy. Reaction time studies, in addition to studies indicating poor coordination and mistiming of the physiology of speech at various levels of the stutterer's production system, suggest a need for the stutterer to take more time to coordinate the complexities of the speech act. Slowing down the speech rate is one therapeutic result.

With regard to the feedback systems, clinicians have found that manipulating the auditory channel may lead to effective fluency control. Both masking and DAF have been used extensively for this purpose. The precise manner in which the two techniques act to reduce stuttering is not known, but masking has been found to increase vocal intensity and, with increased masking intensity, to lengthen syllables and reduce rate of speech. DAF also results in increased vocal intensity and slowed speech rate (see Wingate's (1976) review for further discussion).

Not long after the appearance of Goldiamond's (1965) important conditioning experiments with DAF, Curlee and Perkins (1969) published details of their "Conversational Rate Control Therapy for Stuttering," which incorporates the use of DAF delivered at a 250-msec delay. The clients were instructed to slow down the speaking rate by prolonging syllables while under DAF. When the criterion for fluency was reached, the DAF was adjusted to 200 msec, and subsequently it was attenuated in 50-msec steps until the clients spoke in a prolonged manner with 0 delay. This technique was combined with other procedures to further reduce stuttering and increase the client's control over rate, and eventually to transfer the newer pattern to different situations.

The fluency-enhancing effects of DAF have encouraged others (e.g., Ingham and Andrews, 1971; Ryan and Van Kirk, 1974; Webster, 1970) to incorporate it into therapy programs. Van Riper uses DAF differently from those advocating fluency-shaping techniques in that he encourages the stutterer, while under DAF, to focus on the proprioception of speech.

Ryan (1971) reported the use of DAF on one 8-year-old child, using delay times that he uses on adult stutterers—that is, beginning with a 250-msec delay and reducing in 50-msec steps to 0 delay. In addition, he reported effective therapy with such a technique on children 7 years old (Ryan, 1979, p. 148). Ryan's therapy is discussed in more detail in Chapter 8.

Electromyographic (EMG) biofeedback can be used to deliver information on speech muscle activity back to the stutterer during speech. The stutterer is able to control a signal (variable tone, VU meter, attenuating light) by reducing the amount of work his muscles are doing during speech, presumably by using tactile and proprioceptive monitoring of the amount of tension in the muscles. Guitar (1975) trained three stutterers to reduce the activity of speech-related muscles during speech, particularly lip and laryngeal muscles, when working with variable tone feedback. The subjects experienced an overall reduction in the rate of stuttering; more focused work was continued with one subject, who learned to reduce muscle activity before stuttering occurred and maintained his gain in fluency for at least 9 months after treatment.

Clinicians' attempts to facilitate easy onsets and loose articulatory contacts, rather than tense, hard onsets of speech and voice, are attempts not only at changing motor patterns but in acquiring a different "feel" of speech. (See Chapter 8, p. 196, for discussion of loose contacts.) Tactile and proprioceptive feedback are changed in such a way that the stutterer learns to recognize that "feel" as the desirable sensation to associate with speech production.

Peripheral Speech Production

This section discusses the respiratory, phonatory, and articulatory/coarticulatory levels of stuttering; the aerodynamics of stuttering; and finally, discoordination of the speech production system. The focus is on adults because the physiology of childhood stuttering—for the most part based on the adult research—is discussed in Chapter 5.

Respiratory Level   Reported anomalies of respiration, such as shallow breathing, oppositional breathing, and irregular breathing patterns, have been examined and found to be prevalent during the stutterer's speech production, but not during quiet breathing. Abnormal breathing patterns seem to be part of the symptomatology of stuttering, then, not part of the stutterer's basic physiology. More recent work, carried out with newer instrumentation, has renewed some researchers' interest in respiration and stuttering. Schilling (1960), for example, found that nearly half his subjects exhibited short, clonic contractions within the normal respiratory pattern of quiet breathing. Metz, Conture, and Colton (1976) found asynchrony between the onset of laryngeal movements and chest wall movements before 70% of stuttered words, but in a study of only two subjects. In fluent word production, the two subjects' movements were the same as that of a nonstuttering control. Myers (1976) found a variety of speech-related respiratory differences in 17 stutterers. Her subjects demonstrated a greater relative increase in breathing rate prior to stuttering compared with fluent utterances when responding to questions, but a smaller relative increase in breathing rate when repeating prerecorded single words. Additionally, the subjects exhibited deeper inhalation and exhalation before stuttered responses compared with fluent responses on the word task, but shallower inhalation and exhalation on the question answering task. Although Myers's findings were not statistically significant, they are of interest because of the marked individual variation among the subjects, and the appearance of physiological reactions before the speech utterance.

There is no evidence that respiratory disturbances cause stuttering. There is, however, evidence that respiratory cycles may be disrupted in a variety of ways, and probably on a highly individual basis, during and before stuttering.

Phonatory Level The speed with which stutterers initiate and terminate phonation in vowel and syllable production was discussed previously in connection with the central nervous system. A related issue, and one that involves coordination and timing of the articulators, including the larynx, is voice onset time (VOT). VOT is a measure of the timing of the onset of voice in relation to the movement of the articulators for the release of a consonant—in particular, stop consonants—for the production of a CV syllable. Comprehensive reviews of stutterers' voice onset and offset time have been offered by Andrews et al. (1983), Bloodstein (1981), Freeman (1979), Starkweather (1982a), St. Louis (1979), and Van Riper (1982). All are agreed that VOT is slower in stutterers, as a group, than in nonstutterers.

In addition to the slower timing of phonatory onset in relation to articulatory movement, physiological studies have given direct information on aberrant vocal fold activity during stutterers' speech production. Two such studies, using EMG, have demonstrated higher activity of the laryngeal muscles during the stuttering, cocontraction of adductor and abductor muscles, and generally asynchronous activity of the vocal folds for the speech segment being produced (Freeman and Ushijima, 1978; Shapiro, 1980). Shapiro found similar aberrations of muscle activity during some utterances that had been judged fluent by experienced listeners. These physiological findings have stimulated a good deal of conjecture regarding the role of the larynx during stuttering, particularly in reference to factors of etiology and remediation. Starkweather (1982a) suggested two potential hypotheses—one (which he prefers) in which the larynx is involved with stuttering, but neither more nor less than the remainder of the vocal tract; and one in which the larynx plays a primary role in generating stuttering, so that other parts of the vocal tract become secondary. After an extensive review of the research, Starkweather opted for the first hypothesis: that the larynx is involved with stuttering, but neither more nor less than the remainder of the vocal tract.

Conture, McCall, and Brewer (1977) used a fiberscope to examine the vocal fold behavior of 10 stutterers during different types of stuttering. They found the following tendencies: for abduction of the glottis to occur with part-word repetitions; for adduction of the glottis to occur with prolongations of sounds; and, in a small sample of broken words, for glottal abduction to occur. According to these findings, the glottis is behaving in a fairly predictable manner for more than half the tokens examined, but in other ways for the remainder of the tokens. That is, there is an inconsistent relationship between laryngeal and articulatory behavior.

In brief, the VOT research carried out on adult stutterers has demonstrated almost uniformly slower VOT's, whereas direct examination of the vocal folds during speech tasks has shown aberrant vocal fold behavior during stuttering moments, and, in some instances during stutterers' fluent utterances. An attempt to match laryngeal behavior with articulatory behavior met with limited success.

Articulatory/Coarticulatory Level   Above the larynx, the stutterer's articulatory efforts may be impaired in a variety of ways. For example, there may be unusual pharyngeal movement during stuttering (Zinkin, 1968), or antagonistic activity of the orbicularis oris and the depressor labii inferior (Ford and Luper, 1975). Shapiro (1980) found tension, poor timing, and nonreciprocity not only in the laryngeal musculature, but also in the superior longitudinal muscle of the tongue and in the orbicularis oris.

Attention has also been paid to the nature of transitions in stutterers' speech production, that is, to the vocal portions into and out of a consonant. Starkweather and Myers (1979) found stutterers to have slower transitions into and out of the fricative /s/ in a token extracted from fluent speech. For plosives, Hand and Luper (1980) found stutterers' transitions to be faster than those of nonstutterers. Zimmermann (1980), on the other hand, found stutterers' transitions to be slower than those of nonstutterers for plosives and for /m/.

Aerodynamics   "Aerodynamics" refers to the force or pressure exerted by air in motion. In the vocal tract, the flow of air from the lungs is manipulated during speech production by variable resistance from articulators such as the vocal folds, soft palate, tongue, and lips. Instrumentation enables the measurement of airflow rates, and this measurement reflects the resistance of the vocal tract. Above-average airflow rates, for example, suggest little resistance; below-average rates reflect much resistance. It is also possible to measure the amount of buildup in certain regions, such as subglottal air pressure and intraoral air pressure.

Hutchinson (1975) delineated seven aerodynamic patterns related to different types of stuttering block. For example, the aerodynamic characteristics for syllable repetition were repeated elevations in intraoral air pressure with successful release and appropriate transitions into subsequent phonetic elements; for a brief prolongation, the aerodynamic characteristics were gradual elevations in intraoral pressure (prolonged rise time). Presumably, the increase in intraoral air pressure during a brief prolongation is due to the momentary immobilizing posture of the articulators for the prolongation, with a subsequent buildup of air pressure in the oral cavity.

During a metronome-paced task, Hutchinson and Navarre (1977) found that airflow rates decreased for stutterers and increased for nonstutterers. During stuttered speech there were a variety of aerodynamic aberrations. Adams, Runyon, and Mallard (1975) found this to be true also for the fluent utterances of stutterers, whether whispered or voiced.

The research on the aerodynamics of stuttered speech suggests that the vocal tract of a stutterer may assume postures that interfere with normal airflow, sometimes creating a backup of air pressure. Both glottal and supraglottal levels may influence airflow rates. Aerodynamic problems also occur in fluent utterances of stutterers, perhaps reflecting widespread influences of stuttering, or "subclinical" stuttering, but not necessarily etiological influences.

"Discoordination" of the Speech Production System   Perkins et al. (1976) and Adams (1974, 1975, 1978) emphasized that for smooth, integrated speech production to occur, the entire vocal tract must function as a synergistic whole. Adams has stressed relaxed, coordinated respiration for speech, timed for an easy onset at the glottis and coordinated with articulatory gestures of the upper vocal tract. There should be no supraglottal buildup of air pressure because of tight valving of the articulators. He believes that the speech production system in stutterers does not function in the ideal, coordinated fashion.

Perkins et al. (1976) also have suggested a discoordination of the respiratory, phonatory, and articulatory systems. They attempted to demonstrate that as the system is reduced in complexity for stutterers (from normally voiced oral reading, to whispered reading, to "lipped" reading without airflow), the rate of stutterers' speech increases because of reduced interference of stuttering.

Stutterers show evidence of a discoordination of the speech production system in that irregularities in the coordination of respiration, phonation, and articulation/coarticulation have been found, and the aerodynamics of speech production, which depend on a coordinated system, may be impaired.

Therapeutic Implications   The discoordination hypothesis represents an attempt to synthesize our knowledge of the workings of the vocal tract in normally fluent speech, and to apply this knowledge to the breakdown that occurs in the fluency of stutterers. The implication is that, rather than working on breathing exercises per se with the stutterer, any breathing anomaly should be treated in concert with, for example, an easy onset of voice at the glottis and loose articulatory contacts of the upper vocal tract. That is, efforts must be made to coordinate this complex system and to have the stutterer make smooth transitions from sound to sound.

To help the coordination of the vocal tract for speech production, writers such as Perkins have suggested reducing the complexity of speech production, so that fewer speech gestures will be required at any given moment. Slowing down the speech rate is the technique usually used to simplify the coordination of the speech production mechanism. This may be done by direct instruction to the stutterer or by using some mechanical means, such as DAF.

Studies of the physiology of the stutterer's speech mechanism and its interactive parts have had more implications for therapy than for theory to date. For the physiological aberrations to have significance with regard to etiological theory, they would have to be present at the onset of stuttering, but this has not yet been established. The kinds of investigation carried out on the adult subjects are, generally speaking, inappropriate for young children.

Genetics

Observations that stuttering tends to run in families have been confirmed by genetic studies reported by Andrews and Harris (1964), Kidd (1977, 1980), and Kidd, Kidd, and Records (1978). This research has also shown that, genetically speaking, female stutterers differ from male stutterers, because females who have become stutterers have inherited the "stuttering" gene from both parents more often than have males. As a consequence they transmit the gene more frequently to their children. This results in females having more stuttering relatives than male stutterers. Also, male relatives of female stutterers incur four times the risk of stuttering as compared with female relatives of female stutterers. Whatever it takes genetically to create stuttering in an individual, a female requires more of it to become a stutterer; males have a lower level or threshold of susceptibility. The precise nature of the "predisposition" has not been determined, although the range of possible genetic transmissions has been narrowed down to two types: the single-locus model and the multifactorial model, both of which include a sex-limiting factor. The information above, in addition to partially clarifying etiological aspects of stuttering, provides an explanation for the preponderance of male stutterers as compared with female stutterers, although a linguistic explanation for this has been proposed (Andrews et al. 1983).

Concordance Research   Howie (1981) recently added information to concordance research on stuttering in twins (Nelson, Hunter, and Walter, 1945), which strongly suggested a genetic factor. "Concordance" refers to the degree to which the same characteristics are shared by monozygotic twins (from one ovum and genetically identical) and dizygotic twins (from two ova and genetically comparable to other siblings).

Howie's careful study contained 16 monozygotic and 13 dizygotic twin pairs, each of which contained at least one stutterer or former stutterer. Results of her study demonstrated that the co-twin of a monozygotic twin has a 77% chance of being a stutterer, and the co-twin of a dizygotic twin has a 32% chance of being a stutterer. Because the sibling of a stutterer has a 20% risk of developing the disorder, Howie's findings have obvious relevance in supporting the genetic theory. However, given the discordant monozygotic twins in Howie's sample, a nongenetic factor is implicated for those stutterers. The reasonable explanation that Howie offers for the higher risk of stuttering in the dizygotic twins than in siblings in the general population is that environmental similarity is even greater for the dizygotic twins. This study, although lending considerable credence to genetic theory as the etiology in many cases of stuttering, simultaneously notes that other factors, presumably environmental, operate to cause stuttering in some instances. Howie was unable to identify specific environmental factors of etiological significance.

Therapeutic Implications   It is possible for stutterers to have genetic histories of varying strengths. The genetic history of a stutterer may or may not be accompanied by psychosocial factors that serve to maintain or worsen the stuttering. It behooves the clinician to get as balanced a picture as possible of the relative strengths of the variables involved, to appropriately counsel the parents of a young stutterer, or to counsel the older stutterer. The child who presents both a strong genetic history and unfavorable environmental circumstances, for example, presents greater complexity therapeutically than one with a genetic history and a supportive and caring environment. Focusing on the "key" issues, as far as they can be ascertained, will help the clinician to direct certain aspects of therapy.

Highlights of the Physiological Factor

The areas reviewed and discussed under "Central Nervous System Function" were general brain function, hemispheric dominance for language and speech, reaction time, and feedback mechanisms. Of these, the reaction time studies showed the most consistent differences between stutterers and nonstutterers, with the former having slower reaction times than the latter. The results of the studies of general brain function and hemispheric dominance equivocate sufficiently to suggest that perhaps there is a subgroup of stutterers for whom CNS function is slightly atypical. If feedback mechanisms have a role in the origins of stuttering, that role has yet to be clarified. Feedback mechanisms have been used effectively, however, in the treatment of stuttering.

Aberrations in the function of the peripheral speech production mechanism may be found at all levels of the system, from the respiratory level through to the coordination of the component parts. Although the differences in the function of the peripheral units of the speech mechanism may result from stuttering, findings of such differences between stutterers and nonstutterers in the fluent utterances of the stutterers stimulate theoretical speculations. We pay more attention to such speculations in Chapter 5.

As a result of the physiological research, many therapies require the stutterer to slow down the rate of speech, thus allowing more time for synchronization of the system.

Research into the genetics of stuttering has recently supported the "constitutional" nature of stuttering in many cases. Further information from brain function studies and studies of the peripheral speech mechanism may help to clarify the way in which the genetic component is manifested.

THE PSYCHOLINGUISTIC FACTOR

The reader is referred to Chapter 4 for details on psycholinguistics and stuttering, which are covered in broad perspective here. There is no tradition of a "psycholinguistic theory" or a "linguistic theory" as there is, for example, for the "cerebral dominance theory." However, the potential relationships among various aspects of language, fluency, and disfluency are many. For instance, one might observe stuttering in relation to the language use of the older stutterer, who is an experienced speaker, versus the child who is still acquiring language on any level or blend of levels from the semantic, syntactic, phonological to the pragmatic, or according to suprasegmental features.

Linguistic Theory in Adults

Dalton and Hardcastle (1976) have proposed a model of fluency that they apply to stuttering and to other communicative disorders where fluency may be affected, such as cluttering, dysarthria, and aphasia. They propose several levels of their model: phonetic transition, grammatical, prosodic, and lexical-semantic. For example, the stutterer may have difficulty in making the smooth transitions from sound to sound on the phonetic transition level. Grammatically, the stuttering may be linked to grammatical junctures—clause onsets, for example, where a natural pause or the use of "fillers" would be used by fluent speakers. The stutterer's blocks, or breaks for inhalation at inappropriate places in the utterance, can interrupt the prosody of the sentence. On the semantic-syntactic level, the various circumlocutions of some stutterers interfere with the meaning of an utterance because a feared word or phrase is replaced with another utterance.

Hamre (1976) suggested a "language systems processing model" of stuttering in which stuttering is associated with two levels: a linguistic level ("language systems") and a psychophysical level ("language processing"). Stuttering, according to the model, is mainly a phonological disorder involving sounds at a segmental level and prosody. There is an interaction of context-sensitive rules pertaining to sounds and situations. In addition, there is an interaction of severity and levels; as severity increases, more areas (e.g., the stutterer's ability to use syntax) are affected. The focus is on motor programming for speech production as a means of understanding stuttering.

Wingate's (1976) review of fluency-enhancing factors, in which he summarized the conditions under which stutterers become fluent, led him to identify stuttering as a prosodic defect. He believes that a stutterer stutters in attempting to make the transition from silence or a speech sound to a stressed syllable. "Stuttering occurs when undulations in the vocal sound are moving toward crests of relative prominence. Stuttering is, then, an intermittent disorder actualizing stress increase" (p. 260).

Dalton and Hardcastle (1976), Hamre (1976), and Wingate (1976) have focused their attention on theoretical models that seek to explain stuttering in the experienced speaker. The theories, therefore, are more appropriate to Bloodstein's "moment of stuttering" than to an etiological theory, although Dalton and Hardcastle evince interest in the acquisition of language in relation to fluency.

Linguistic Theory in Children

Many recent studies seek to explain the relation of early stuttering to linguistic variables (see Chapter 4). Some relate specifically to stutterers, and some pertain to the nonfluencies of normally speaking youngsters. The research focuses on the following areas: the rate of language acquisition of young stutterers as compared with nonstutterers, clinical observations that some young language-delayed children in therapy develop stuttering or stuttering-like symptoms, an apparent relation between the nonfluencies of highly nonfluent youngsters and stutterers and a reduction in their use of syntactic complexity, the appearance of transient nonfluencies in normally fluent children with the appearance of new semantic-syntactic structures, and the distribution of stuttering according to the constituent structure of an utterance.

The language area that has received most exploration to date is rate of language acquisition in young stutterers. Andrews et al. (1983) cite six studies that confirm the delay and one that does not. They conclude that the delay in language acquisition in stutterers averages about 6 months. They also refer to eight studies confirming linguistic deficits of various kinds in childhood stutterers; tests such as the Peabody Picture Vocabulary Test, length and complexity of utterance, and subtests of the Illinois Tests of Psycholinguistic Abilities were used in the studies. In addition, they cite seven studies demonstrating that stutterers are three times more at risk of articulation disorder than are nonstutterers.

Studies examining the loci of stuttering in the speech of young stutterers in relation to constituent structure have also demonstrated that the point of breakdown for the youngster is related to clause onsets (Bernstein, 1981; Wall, Starkweather, and Cairns, 1981) or clause and phrase onsets (Bloodstein, 1974; Bloodstein and Grossman, 1981). The phenomenon of clause onset stuttering is of interest because at this point in the utterance a variety of cognitive and physiological events are taking place. It is thought to be the point at which sentence planning occurs (Fodor, Bever, and Garrett, 1974; Garrett, 1976) and it is the point at which respiration usually takes place for fluent speech and where phonation is initiated—a complex moment in the sentence.

Language-delayed Children   Stuttering typically begins in the language-learning years, and one might reasonably hypothesize some linguistic stress on the entire system of language planning and speech production of the delayed youngster. And the stress of language acquisition may continue longer than we have suspected. Ingram (1975), for example, claims that the major development in the child's ability to produce sentence complexity in the form of embeddedness occurs after 6 years of age. Before that, the child may use relative clauses that are part of stock phrases, but true sentence complexity emerges later. Limber (1973) traced the beginnings of sentence complexity to less than 3 years of age. Ingram's point is, however, that mature use of complexity arrives later. We are not suggesting that linguistic complexity causes stuttering in the child who begins to stutter after entering school. But, given what has been observed regarding fluency and language acquisition, it is worth considering as a factor along with better known factors—such as genetics and environmental influences. Even the mildly language-delayed child might be more vulnerable to breakdown at times of significant language acquisition, such as complexity.

Not all stutterers, of course, are language delayed. It is appropriate, however, to contemplate a theory that includes a genetic factor that might result in a slightly incoordinated motor apparatus for speech production, which, in concert with the linguistic stress of language delay, could account for the breakdown in the speech of many youngsters. The sites of breakdown in the utterance would logically be the more vulnerable points where linguistic and physiological processes are at work for the next part of the utterance, that is, the clause boundaries. This theory could also account for children without language delay, who, given the genetic under-pinnings of stuttering and potentially poorly coordinated speech muscula-ture, would also logically break down at clause boundaries, where the physiological processes for respiration and the initiation of speech and voice take place.

Therapeutic Implications   There are some common-sense implications of psycholinguistic theory for the older stutterer whose language is already advanced. The stutterer needs to observe, for example, appropriate clause boundary pauses to maintain the melody of speech and to facilitate sentence planning. In addition, he or she needs to maintain the integrity of the clause so that the listener will be able to perceive the statement correctly (Fodor, Bever, and Garrett, 1974). Inhalation for speech, therefore, must occur before the onset of the clause (or at least the phrase), not at inappropriate midpoints, or midword.

Wingate (1976) has made direct application of his theory of "stress actualization" to therapy, and he includes methods such as singing and Froeschel's voice chewing to encourage stutterers to vocalize easily. Further instruction includes helping the client to develop the melody of speech and efficient use of linguistic stress.

For the young child, the interest in language as a part of the fluency disorder has led to the development of language-based therapies. Such therapies are exemplified by the Stocker probe (1980), Gregory and Hill's (1980) therapy, and, in part, by our own therapy. Because children are usually fluent on very short utterances, and are likely to be disfluent on longer and complex utterances, clinicians have been encouraged to use language structure as a method of facilitating fluency.

Highlights of the Psycholinguistic Factor

The psycholinguistic factor may be applied to the advanced stutterer and to the child stutterer to aid in describing or understanding the moment of stuttering. For the beginning speaker, language is part of a complex array of developing skills, many of which contribute to fluency. A breakdown in a component or components may disrupt normal language and speech acquisition and result in stuttering. The smooth integration of linguistic and speech motor skills is thought to be essential to fluent speech. Therapy programs for young stutterers are increasingly acknowledging the psycho-linguistic component and its influence on fluency.

REFERENCES

Adams, M. R. 1974. Vocal tract dynamics in fluency and stuttering: A review and interpretation of past research. In: L. M. Webster and L. C. Furst (eds.), Vocal Tract Dynamics and Dysfluency, pp. 10–28. Speech and Hearing Institute, New York.

Adams, M. R. 1975. Letter to the editor. J. Speech Hear. Disord. 40:136.

Adams, M. R. 1978. Stuttering theory, research, therapy: The present and future. J. Fluency Disord. 3:139–147.

Adams, M. R. 1980. The young stutterer: Diagnosis, treatment and assessment of progress. Semin. Speech Lang. Hear. 1:289–300.

Adams, M. R., and Moore, W. M., Jr. 1972. The effects of auditory masking on the anxiety level, frequency of dysfluency, and selected vocal characteristics of stutterers. J. Speech Hear. Res. 15:572–578.

Adams, M. R., Runyon, C., and Mallard, A. R. 1975. Airflow characteristics of the speech of stutterers and nonstutterers. J. Fluency Disord. 1:3–12.

Andrews, G., Craig, A., Feyer, A. M., Hoddinott, S., Howie, P., and Neilson, M. 1983. Stuttering: A review of research findings circa 1982. J. Speech Hear. Disord. 48:226–246.

Andrews, G., and Harris, M. 1964. The Syndrome of Stuttering. Clinics in Developmental Medicine, no. 17. Spastics Society Medical Education and Information Unit in association with William Heinemann, Medicine Books, London.

Barbara, D. A. 1954. Stuttering: A Psychodynamic Approach to Its Understanding and Treatment. Julian Press, New York.

Barbara, D. A. 1965. New Directions in Stuttering: Theory and Practice. Charles C Thomas Publisher, Springfield, Ill.

Bernstein, N. 1981. Are there constraints on childhood disfluency? J. Fluency Disord. 6:341–350.

Bloodstein, O. 1958. Stuttering as an anticipatory struggle reaction. In: J. Eisenson (ed.), Stuttering: A Symposium, pp.1–69. Harper & Row, New York.

Bloodstein, O. 1972. The anticipatory struggle hypothesis: Implications of research on the variability of stuttering. J. Speech Hear. Res. 15:487–499.

Bloodstein, O. 1974. The rules of early stuttering. J. Speech Hearing Disord. 39:379–394.

Bloodstein, O. 1975. Stuttering as tension and fragmentation. In: J. Eisenson (ed.), Stuttering: A Second Symposium, pp.1–95. Harper & Row, New York.

Bloodstein, O. 1981. A Handbook on Stuttering. 3rd Ed. National Easter Seal Society, Chicago.

Bloodstein, O., and Grossman, M. 1981. Early stutterings: Some aspects of their form and distribution. J. Speech Hear. Res. 24:298–302.

Borden, G. J. 1979. An interpretation of research on feedback interruption in speech. Brain Lang. 7:307–319.

Borden, G. J., and Harris, K. S. 1980. Speech Science Primer: Physiology, Acoustics and Perception of Speech. Williams & Wilkins Company, Baltimore.

Brutten, E. J., and Shoemaker, D. J. 1967. The Modification of Stuttering. Prentice-Hall, Englewood Cliffs, N.J.

Cerf, A., and Prins, D. 1974. Stutterers' ear preference for dichotic syllables. Paper presented at the American Speech and Hearing Association Convention, Las Vegas.

Chase, R. A., Sutton, S., First, D., and Zubin, J. 1961. A developmental study of changes in behavior under delayed auditory feedback. J. Genet. Psychol. 99:101–112.

Cherry, C., and Sayers, B. 1956. Experiments upon the total inhibition of stammering by external control and some clinical results. J. Psychosom. Res. 1:233–246.

Cimorell-Strong, J. M., Gilbert, H. R., and Frick, J. V. 1983. Dichotic speech perception: A comparison between stuttering and nonstuttering children. J. Fluency Disord. 8:77–91.

Colburn, N., and Mysak, E. D. 1982. Developmental disfluency and emerging grammar. II. Co-occurrence of disfluency with specified semantic-syntactic structures. J. Speech Hear. Res. 25:421–427.

Conture, E. G. 1974. Some effects of noise on the speaking behavior of stutterers. J. Speech Hear. Res. 17:714–723.

Conture, E., McCall, G., and Brewer, D. 1977. Laryngeal behavior during stuttering. J. Speech Hear. Res. 20:661–668.

Cooper, E. B. 1975. Clinicians' attitudes toward stutterers: A study of bigotry? Paper presented at the American Speech and Hearing Association Convention, Washington, D.C.

Cooper, E. B. 1979. Intervention procedures for the young stutterer. In: H. H. Gregory (ed.), Controversies About Stuttering Therapy, pp. 63–96. University Park Press, Baltimore.

Coriat, I. H. 1927. The oral-erotic components of stammering. Int. J. Psychoanal. 8:56–69.

Coriat, I. H. 1931. The nature and analytic treatment of stuttering. Proc. Am. Speech Correction Assoc. 1:151–156.

Coriat, I. H. 1943. The psychoanalytic concept of stammering. Nerv. Child. 2:167–171.

Costello, J. 1975. The establishment of fluency with time-out procedures: Three case studies. J. Speech Hear. Disord. 40:216–231.

Costello, J. 1980. Operant conditioning and the treatment of stuttering. Semin. Speech, Lang. Hear. 1:311–326.

Cullen, J. K., Fargo, N., Chase, R. A., and Baker, P. 1968. The development of auditory feedback monitoring: Delayed auditory feedback studies on infant cry. J. Speech Hear. Res. 11:85–93.

Curlee, R. F., and Perkins, W. H. 1969. Conversational rate control therapy for stuttering. J. Speech Hear. Disord. 34:245–250.

Curry, F. K. W., and Gregory, H. H. 1969. The performance of stutterers on dichotic listening tasks thought to reflect cerebral dominance. J. Speech Hear. Res. 12:72–82.

Dalton, P., and Hardcastle, W. J. 1976. Disorders of Fluency and Their Effects on Communication. Elsevier North-Holland, New York.

Daly, D. A., and Cooper, E. B. 1967. Rate of stuttering adaptation under two electro-shock conditions. Behav. Res. Ther. 5:49–54.

Daly, D. A., and Frick, J. V. 1970. The effects of punishing stuttering expectations and stuttering utterances: A comparative study. Behav. Ther. 1:228–239.

Fenichel, O. 1945. The Psychoanalytic Theory of Neurosis. W. W. Norton, New York.

Fodor, J. A., Bever, T. G., and Garrett, M. F. 1974. The Psychology of Language. McGraw-Hill Book Company, New York.

Ford, S., and Luper, H. 1975. Aerodynamic, phonatory, and labial EMG patterns during fluent and stuttered speech. Paper presented at the American Speech and Hearing Association Convention, Washington, D.C.

Freeman, F. J. 1979. Phonation in stuttering: A review of current research. J. Fluency Disord. 4:78–89.

Freeman, F., and Ushijima, T. 1978. Laryngeal muscle activity during stuttering. J. Speech Hear. Res. 21:538–562.

Frick, J. V. 1970. Motor Planning Techniques for the Treatment of Stuttering. Manuscript. Pennsylvania State University, University Park.

Garrett, M. F. 1976. Syntactic processes in sentence production. In: R. J. Wales and E. Walker (eds.), New Approaches to Language Mechanisms, pp. 231–256. Elsevier North-Holland, New York.

Glauber, I. P. 1958. The psychoanalysis of stuttering. In: J. Eisenson (ed.), Stuttering: A Symposium, pp. 71–119. Harper & Row, New York.

Goldiamond, I. 1965. Stuttering and fluency as manipulatable operant response classes. In: L. Krasner and L. P. Ullman (eds.), Research in Behavior Modification, pp. 106–156. Holt Rinehart & Winston, New York.

Gregory, H. H., and Hill, D. 1980. Stuttering therapy for children. Semin. Speech, Lang. Hear. 1:351–364.

Gruber, L., and Powell, R. L. 1974. Responses of stuttering and nonstuttering children to a dichotic listening task. Percept. Motor Skills. 38:203–204.

Guitar, B. 1975. Reduction of stuttering frequency using analog electromyographic feedback. J. Speech Hear. Res. 18:672–685.

Guitar, B. E., Kopff, H., Kilburg, G. D., and Conway, P. 1981. Parental verbal interactions and speech rate: A case study in stuttering. Paper presented at the American Speech-Language-Hearing Association, Los Angeles.

Hamre, C. 1976. Stuttering: A language systems and processing model. Paper presented at the American Speech and Hearing Association Convention, Houston.

Hand, C. R., and Luper, H. L. 1980. Durational characteristics of stutterers' and nonstutterers' fluent speech. A.S.H.A. 22(abstr.):709.

Hannley, M., and Dorman, M. F. 1982. Some observations on auditory function and stuttering. J. Fluency Disord. 7:93–108.

Haroldson, S. K., Martin, R. R., and Starr, C. D. 1968. Time-out as a punishment for stuttering. J. Speech Hear. Res. 11:560–566.

Heilpern, E. 1941. A case of stuttering. Psychoanal. Q. 1:95–115.

Helm, N. A., Butler, R. B., and Canter, G. J. 1980. Neurogenic acquired stuttering. J. Fluency Disord. 5:269–279.

Howie, P. M. 1981. Concordance for stuttering in monozygotic and dizygotic twin pairs. J. Speech Hear. Res. 24:317–321.

Hutchinson, J. M. 1975. Aerodynamic patterns of stuttered speech. In: L. M. Webster and L. C. Furst (eds.), Vocal Tract Dynamics and Dysfluency, pp. 71–110. Speech and Hearing Institute, New York.

Hutchinson, J. M., and Navarre, B. M. 1977. The effect of metronome pacing on selected aerodynamic patterns of stuttered speech: Some preliminary observations and interpretations. J. Fluency Disord. 2:189–206.

Hutchinson, J. M., and Ringel, R. L. 1975. The effect of oral sensory deprivation on stuttering behavior. J. Commun. Disord. 8:249–258.

Ingham, R. J., and Andrews, G. 1971. Stuttering: The quality of fluency after treatment. J. Commun. Disord. 4:279–288.

Ingram, D. 1975. If and when transformations are acquired by children. In: D. P. Dato (ed.), Georgetown University Round Table on Languages and Linguistics 1975, pp. 99–127. Georgetown University Press, Washington, D.C.

Johnson, L. J. 1980. Facilitating parental involvement in the therapy of the disfluent child. Semin. Speech Lang. Hear. 1:301–309.

Johnson, W. 1955. A study of the onset and development of stuttering. In: W. Johnson and R. R. Leutenegger (eds.), Stuttering in Children and Adults, pp. 37–73. University of Minnesota Press, Minneapolis.

Johnson, W., and Associates. 1959. The Onset of Stuttering. University of Minnesota Press, Minneapolis.

Kidd, K. K. 1977. A genetic perspective on stuttering. J. Fluency Disord. 2:259–269.

Kidd, K. K. 1980. Genetic models of stuttering. J. Fluency Disord. 5:187–202.

Kidd, K. K., Kidd, J. R., and Records, M. A. 1978. The possible causes of the sex ratio in stuttering and its implications. J. Fluency Disord. 3:13–23.

Lee, B. S. 1950. Effects of delayed speech feedback. J. Acoust. Soc. Am. 22:824–826.

Lee, B. S. 1951. Artificial stutter. J. Speech Hear. Disord. 16:53–55.

Limber, J. 1973. The genesis of complex sentences. In: T. Moore (ed.), Cognitive Development and the Acquisition of Language, pp. 171–185. Academic Press, New York.

Mackay, D. G. 1968. Metamorphosis of a critical interval: Age-linked changes in the delay in auditory feedback that produces maximal disruption of speech. J. Acoust. Soc. Am. 43:811–821.

Maraist, J. A., and Hutton, C. 1957. Effects of auditory masking upon the speech of stutterers. J. Speech Hear. Disord. 22:385–389.

Martin, R. R., and Haroldson, S. K. 1971. Time-out as a punishment for stuttering during conversation. J. Commun. Disord. 4:15–19.

Martin, R. R., Kuhl, P., and Haroldson, S. 1972. An experimental treatment with two preschool stuttering children. J. Speech Hear. Res. 15:743–752.

Metz, D. E., Conture, E. G., and Colton, R. H. 1976. Temporal relations between the respiratory and laryngeal systems prior to stuttered disfluencies. Paper presented at the American Speech and Hearing Association Convention, Houston.

Moore, W. H., Jr., and Haynes, W. O. 1980. Alpha hemispheric asymmetry and stuttering: Some support for a segmentation dysfunction hypothesis. J. Speech Hear. Res. 23:229–247.

Moore, W. H., Jr., and Lang, M. K. 1977. Alpha asymmetry over the right and left hemispheres of stutterers and control subjects preceding massed oral readings: A preliminary investigation. Percep. Motor Skills. 44:223–230.

Moore, W. H., Jr., and Lorendo, L. C. 1980. Hemispheric alpha asymmetries of stuttering males and nonstuttering males and females for words of high and low imagery. J. Fluency Disord. 5:11–26.

Myers, F. L. 1976. Physiological correlates immediately prior to speech for stutterers and nonstutterers. Unpublished doctoral dissertation. Pennsylvania State University, University Park.

Neelley, J. N. 1961. A study of the speech behavior of stutterers and nonstutterers under normal and delayed auditory feedback. J. Speech Hear. Disord. Monog. Suppl. 7:63–82.

Nelson, S. E., Hunter, N., and Walter, M. 1945. Stuttering in twin types. J. Speech Disord. 10:335–343.

Orton, S. T. 1927. Studies in stuttering. Arch. Neurol. Psychiatr. 18:671–672.

Perkins, W., Rudas, J., Johnson, L., and Bell, J. 1976. Stuttering: Discoordination of phonation with articulation and respiration. J. Speech Hear. Res. 19:509–522.

Perrin, K. L., and Eisenson, J. 1970. An examination of ear preference for speech and nonspeech stimuli in a stuttering population. Paper presented at the American Speech and Hearing Association Convention, New York.

Prosek, R. A., Montgomery, A. A., Walden, B. E., and Schwartz, D. M. 1979.

Reaction-time measures of stutterers and nonstutterers. J. Fluency Disord. 4:269–278.

Quinn, P. T. 1972. Cerebral dominance and the dichotic word test. Med. J. Aust. 2:639–643.

Reed, C. G., and Godden, A. L. 1977. An experimental treatment using verbal punishment with two preschool stutterers. J. Fluency Disord. 2:225–233.

Rieber, R. W., and Wollock, J. 1977. The historical roots of theory and therapy of stuttering. In: R. W. Rieber (ed.), The Problems of Stuttering: Theory and Therapy, pp. 3–24. Elsevier North-Holland, New York.

Rosenfield, D. B., and Goodglass, H. 1980. Dichotic testing of cerebral dominance in stutterers. Brain Lang. 11:170–180.

Ryan, B. P. 1971. Operant procedures applied to stuttering therapy for children. J. Speech Hear. Disord. 36:264–280.

Ryan, B. P. 1974. Programmed Therapy for Stuttering in Children and Adults. Charles C Thomas Publishers, Springfield, Ill.

Ryan, B. P. 1979. Stuttering therapy in a framework of operant conditioning and programmed learning. In: H. H. Gregory (ed.), Controversies About Stuttering Therapy, pp. 129–173. University Park Press, Baltimore.

Ryan, B., and Van Kirk, B. 1974. The establishment, transfer, and maintenance of fluent speech in 50 stutterers using delayed auditory feedback and operant procedures. J. Speech Hear. Disord. 39:3–10.

Schilling, A. 1960. Röntgen-Zwerchfell-kymogramme bei stotterern. Fol. Phoniatr. 12:145–153.

Shames, G. H., and Sherrick, C. E., Jr. 1963. A discussion of nonfluency and stuttering as operant behavior. J. Speech Hear. Disord. 28:3–18.

Shane, M. L. S. 1955. Effect on stuttering of alteration in auditory feedback. In: W. Johnson and R. R. Leutenegger (eds.), Stuttering in Children and Adults, pp. 286–297. University of Minnesota Press, Minneapolis.

Shapiro, A. 1980. An electromyographic analysis of the fluent and dysfluent utterance of several types of stutterers. J. Fluency Disord. 5:203–231.

Sheehan, J. G. 1953. Theory and treatment of stuttering as an approach-avoidance conflict. J. Psychol. 36:27–49.

Sheehan, J. G. 1958. Conflict theory of stuttering. In: J. Eisenson (ed.), Stuttering: A Symposium, pp. 121–166. Harper & Row, New York.

Siegel, G. M., Fehst, C. A., Garber, S. R., and Pick, H. L. 1980. Delayed auditory feedback with children. J. Speech Hear. Res. 23:802–813.

Slorach, N., and Noehr, B. 1973. Dichotic listening in stuttering and dyslalic children. Cortex. 9:295–300.

Sommers, R. K., Brady, W. A., and Moore, W. H., Jr. 1975. Dichotic ear preferences of stuttering children and adults. Percept. Motor Skills. 41:931–938.

Starkweather, C. W. 1982a. Stuttering and Laryngeal Behavior: A Review. American Speech-Language Hearing Association Monographs, no. 21.

Starkweather, C. W. 1982b. Speech and Language: Principles and Processes of Behavior Change. Prentice-Hall, Englewood Cliffs, N.J.

Starkweather, C., and Myers, M. 1979. Duration of subsegments within the intervocalic interval in stutterers and nonstutterers. J. Fluency Disord. 4:205–214.

St. Louis, K. O. 1979. Linguistic and motor aspects of stuttering. In: N. Lass (ed.) , Speech and Language: Advances in Basic Research and Practice; pp. 89–210. Vol. 1. Academic Press, New York.

St. Louis, K. O., and Lass, N. J. 1981. A survey of communicative disorders students' attitudes towards stuttering. J. Fluency Disord. 6:49–80.

Stocker, B. 1980. The Stocker Probe Technique: For Diagnosis and Treatment of Stuttering in Young Children. Modern Education Corporation, Tulsa.

Stromsta, C. 1956. A methodology related to the determination of the phase angle of bone-conducted speech sound energy of stutterers and nonstutterers. Unpublished doctoral dissertation. Ohio State University, Columbus.

Stromsta, C. 1959. Experimental blockage of phonation by distorted sidetone. J. Speech Hear. Res. 2:286–301.

Stromsta, C. 1972. Interaural phase disparity of stutterers and nonstutterers. J. Speech Hear. Res. 15:771–780.

Timmons, B., and Boudreau, J. 1978. Delayed auditory feedback and the speech of stuttering and non-stuttering children. Percept. Motor Skills. 46:551–555.

Travis, L. E. 1931. Speech Pathology. Prentice-Hall, Englewood Cliffs, N.J.

Travis, L. E. 1971. The unspeakable feelings of people with special reference to stuttering. In: L. E. Travis (ed.), Handbook of Speech Pathology and Audiology, pp. 1009–1033. Appleton-Century-Crofts, New York.

Van Riper, C. 1958. Experiments in stuttering therapy. In: J. Eisenson (ed.), Stuttering: A Symposium, pp. 273–390. Harper & Row, New York.

Van Riper, C. 1963. Speech Correction: Principles and Methods. 4th Ed. Prentice-Hall, Englewood Cliffs, N.J.

Van Riper, C. 1971. The Nature of Stuttering. Prentice-Hall, Englewood Cliffs, N.J.

Van Riper, C. 1973. The Treatment of Stuttering. Prentice-Hall, Englewood Cliffs, N.J.

Van Riper, C. 1982. The Nature of Stuttering. 2nd Ed. Prentice-Hall, Englewood Cliffs, N.J.

Wall, M. J., Starkweather, C. W., and Cairns, H. S. 1981. Syntactic influences on stuttering in young child stutterers. J. Fluency Disord. 6:283–298.

Webster, R. L. 1970. Stuttering: A way to eliminate it and a way to explain it. In: R. Ulrich, T. Stachnik, and J. Mabry (eds.), Control of Human Behavior, pp. 157–160, Vol. 2. Scott, Foresman, Glenview, Ill.

Webster, R. L. 1974. A behavioral analysis of stuttering: Treatment and theory. In: K. S. Calhoun, H. E. Adams, and K. M. Mitchell (eds.), Innovative Treatment Methods in Psychopathology, pp. 17–61. John Wiley & Sons, New York.

Webster, R. L. 1977. Concept and theory in stuttering: An insufficiency of empiricism. In: R. W. Rieber (ed.), The Problems of Stuttering: Theory and Therapy, pp. 65–71. Elsevier North-Holland, New York.

Webster, R. L. 1979. Empirical considerations regarding stuttering therapy. In: H. H. Gregory (ed.), Controversies About Stuttering Therapy, pp. 209–239. University Park Press, Baltimore.

Webster, R. L., and Dorman, M. F. 1971. Changes in reliance on auditory feedback cues as a function of oral practice. J. Speech Hear. Res. 14:307–311.

Wiener, N. 1948. Cybernetics. Sci. Am. 179:14–19.

Wingate, M. E. 1976. Stuttering: Theory and Treatment. Irvington Publishers, New York.

Wolpe, J. 1958. Psychotherapy by Reciprocal Inhibition. Stanford University Press, Stanford, Calif.

Yates, A. J. 1963. Delayed Auditory Feedback. Psychol. Bul. 60:213–232.

Yeni-Komshian, G., Chase, R. A., and Mobley, R. L. 1968. The development of auditory feedback monitoring: 11. Delayed auditory feedback studies on the speech of children between two and three years of age. J. Speech Hear. Res. 11:307–315.

Zimmermann, G. 1980. Articulatory dynamics of fluent utterances of stutterers and nonstutterers. J. Speech Hear. Res. 23:95–107.

Zinkin, N. I. 1968. Mechanisms of Speech. Mouton, the Hague, the Netherlands.

3
Symptomatology of Childhood Stuttering

One of the more challenging tasks in the study of stuttering is arriving at a comprehensive yet behaviorally specific definition of stuttering. We concur with Bloodstein's view that although stuttering can be defined generally as excessive or abnormal disruptions in the rhythm or fluency of speech, it may be more fruitful to speak of stuttering in terms of specific disfluency behaviors, such as syllable repetitions or sound prolongations. The primacy of sound and syllable repetitions and prolongations, whether audible or inaudible, is highlighted in Wingate's (1964) definition of stuttering. The latter is reinforced by Andrews et al. (1983): "While this is not a fact there is a consensus that repetitions and prolongations are necessary and sufficient for the diagnosis of stuttering to be made" (p. 227).

INCIDENCE AND PREVALENCE

Incidence and prevalence figures are quantitative indices of the degree of occurrence of a phenomenon. Aside from the purely statistical interest these figures bear, incidence and prevalence data also shed insight into the nature of stuttering.

Incidence is an index, usually expressed as a percentage or the number of individuals in a thousand, indicating the relative number of individuals in a population who have ever stuttered. A wide range of incidence figures exists and this variability can be attributed to differences in the populations studied (including cultural differences across or within a population), in the localities from which the samples were drawn, in the methods of collecting data, in the sizes of samples studied, and in the parameters that were used to define stuttering. The method of data collection, for example, can consist of a longitudinal or a cross-sectional survey of incidence figures in a population; data can be collected by surveying the stutterers themselves or through interviews with parents. The ideal approach would be a longitudinal study in which children's speech are sampled and analyzed over the course of months or years.

Incidence figures range from a low of 0.93% (Cooper, Parris, and Wells, 1974) in a survey of more than 7,000 college freshmen, to a high of 15.4% in a study by Glasner and Rosenthal (1957) of nearly 1,000 first graders. Most such studies have been cross-sectional. One of the few large scale, longitudinal studies of developmental stuttering is the Newcastle-upon-Tyne study by Andrews and Harris (1964) of more than 1,000 children who were followed longitudinally from birth to 16 years of age. One of the disadvantages of longitudinal studies is the high attrition rate through the years, and the study by Andrews and Harris is no exception.

By the end of the study, the original sample of 1,142 children had been reduced to 750 children by "deaths and removals." Nonetheless, this study yielded some valuable data on incidence and prevalence figures for a large group of children in an industrial city in England. The incidence figure was around 3% for the children whose stuttering lasted for 6 months or more, but was 4.5% when those whose stuttering was more transient were included. The onset of stuttering occurred mostly before 5 years of age for the children sampled, and no stutterers had an onset beyond 11 years of age.

Prevalence figures indicate the number of stutterers found at a specific time for a specific population. As with incidence data, prevalence statistics vary depending on the type of population studied, the ages of subjects sampled, and the method of data collection. It is generally agreed that the prevalence of stuttering declines gradually as a function of increasing age, especially toward the high school grades. It is also generally agreed that the prevalence figure for stuttering in prepubertal school children is approximately 1%.

Incidence and prevalence figures become even more revealing when broken down in terms of sex, age of onset of the stuttering, and other accompanying speech and language problems. Brady and Hall (1976), for example, found the sex ratio of 3.9 boys to 1 girl based on a sample of kindergarteners to twelfth graders, most of whom were of normal, but some of whom were of low intelligence. Gillespie and Cooper (1973) found a sex ratio of 2.7 boys to 1 girl in their sample of seventh through twelfth graders. In their comprehensive state-of-the-art paper, Andrews et al. (1983) posed some summary statements regarding our knowledge of stuttering. One such statement noted that three times as many boys as girls stutter and this ratio increases with age. An exception to the foregoing sex differentials consists of some preliminary data based on parent perception for 22 stutterers aged 2 and 3 years (Yairi, 1983). The distribution was similar for boys and girls, and Yairi suggests that the larger sex ratios reported in earlier studies for older children "reflect earlier and/or higher ratio of spontaneous recovery among females" (p. 177). Other conjectures range from a genetic predisposition to stuttering for boys (e.g., Kidd, Kidd, and Records, 1978), to varying sets of social demands and expectations made on boys as compared to girls. In addition to sex differentials based on studies of children from different families, statistics on the incidence of stuttering within families also point to the possibility of a genetic predisposition, although environmental factors cannot be discounted. Andrews and Harris (1964), for example, found a higher percentage of stutterers whose family member(s) also stuttered, compared to the general population.

Many of the data regarding age of onset have been based on parental reports. The variables that influence the validity and reliability of clinical judgment made by a speech-language pathologist should, of course, also be considered when examining data based on parental judgments of normal versus pathological disfluencies. These variables include the parents' definition of stuttering, the intermittency of stuttering during its early stages, and remission or "self-recovery" of early stuttering (Van Riper, 1982, pp. 32–33). For lack of any other source of information regarding the initial periods during the onset of stuttering, we often must rely on recollections by parents or by the stutterers themselves.

The consensus drawn from the literature is that stuttering usually begins during the preschool years, with a gradual decline in onset as a function of increasing age. Onset of stuttering during late childhood or adulthood is rare except in cases of brain injury (e.g., Canter, 1971; Helm, Butler, and Canter, 1980). The earliest age of stuttering onset occurs around 1.5 to 2 years of age, although the most prominent peak of onset occurs around 3 to 4 years of age (Dickson, 1971; Johnson and Associates, 1959). Perhaps not coincidentally, these are also the formative years of speech and language development. Chapter 4 discusses some possible relations between fluency and speech-language development that may account for the covariation between the latter and the peak period for onset of stuttering during early childhood.

BEHAVIORAL DIMENSIONS OF STUTTERING

Introductory Note

Although the term "behavioral" has come to mean "observable behavior" to recent generations of speech-language clinicians, it is used here in its broadest sense to include a wide range of human responses. The spectrum covers the covert as well as overt responses of the psychosocial, physiological, and psycholinguistic factors, and the interactions among them. Adopting a broadly based approach to the clinical management of childhood stuttering necessitates looking at the surface manifestations of disfluencies, such as sound prolongations, as well as the embedded affective components and physiological correlates of stuttering. To consider only the "observable" behaviors of a young stutterer would abort an otherwise more thorough examination of the child's disfluencies.

Complexity of the Moment of Stuttering

There are various schemas for examining stuttering behaviors. Van Riper (1982), for example, dichotomizes stuttering behaviors into the overt features and the covert, affective reactions experienced by stutterers. Most of the affective reactions characterize "stuttering in its full-fledged form." Much of early stuttering is characterized primarily by syllable repetitions and sound prolongations. Early stuttering is also characterized by episodicity and the relative lack of tension and fear. However, the possibility that some of the very young stutterers also show tension, fear, and accessory characteristics cannot be precluded. For a detailed discussion of the onset and development of early stuttering, see the section on "Development of Stuttering" in this chapter.

Van Riper views the overt features of stuttering as "attempts to search for the integrations that will make the utterance of the word possible" (Van Riper, 1982, p. 112). Certain patterns usually can be gleaned from the array of overt behaviors, even though the symptomatology of stuttering is vast and diverse. To impose some organizational framework on the nearly infinite varieties of behavior exhibited by stutterers, the core behavior is differentiated from the accessory or secondary features of stuttering.[1] The core features consist of repetitions, and prolongations or tonic fixations. The latter can be audible or silent as in tense pauses. Prolongations have been observed to develop later than repetitions in many stutterers. Due to the phonetic nature of sounds, audible prolongations occur often on vowels and continuants, and the inaudible fixations of an articulatory or laryngeal posture occur often on CV or CVC syllables beginning with plosives. In the latter instances, the stutterer has difficulty initiating speech at the supralaryngeal level, at the laryngeal level, or both. These blockages or closures have also been referred to in the literature as "tense pauses."

We use the term "tense pause" to mean the inaudible fixations or blockages experienced as a core feature of stuttering. In the sense that the tense pauses are silent and prolonged fixations of the articulatory/laryngeal posture, according to Van Riper, these core symptoms belong to the category of prolongations.

The reader should be aware of the varying terminologies in the literature, particularly in reference to "pause." Some authors have designated pauses as "filled" or "unfilled," at least in reference to normal speakers (Starkweather, 1980), "grammatical" or "ungrammatical" (Dejoy and Gregory, 1975), "conventional" or "idiosyncratic" (Henderson, Goldman-

---

[1]Various classification systems exist for describing stuttering behaviors. In isolated instances, ambiguities may result from attempts to compare one system of classification to another. A term may be used by one author to refer to a specific type of behavior whereas another writer may use the term generically to name a broader class of behaviors. Nonetheless, there is general agreement that the basic essence of stuttering can be classified as repetitions, prolongations, and tense pauses. These behaviors have been referred to as "core behaviors" by Van Riper (1982), and "elemental characteristics" of stuttering by Wingate (1964). The remaining symptoms have been referred to as "associated symptoms" by Bloodstein (1981), "accessory behaviors" by Wingate (1964), and "accessory" (i.e., not basic) or "secondary" (i.e., occurring later in development) features by Van Riper (1982).

Eisler, and Skarbek, 1966), and "tense" pauses. Colburn and Mysak (1982a), for example, used a classification system based on Johnson's unpublished, revised schema in which Johnson added the categories of disrhythmic phonation and tension but omitted the categories of broken words and prolongations. In particular, disrhythmic phonations consist of within-word phonatory distortions that disrupt the flow of speech. Disrhythmic phonations can be but are not necessarily accompanied by tension; they include but are not limited to prolonged sounds, unusual stress or timing, and breaks. The category of tense pause (or simply "tension") was used to refer to barely audible manifestations of heavy breathing or muscular tension existing "between words, part-words, and nonwords like interjections."

Accessory or secondary stuttering can be manifested in a great many and individualistic ways. These accessory behaviors are learned primarily through operant conditioning and evolve through time, either as reactions to the experience of repetitions and prolongations or to the fear of having repetitions and prolongations. Reactions to the experience of prolongations and repetitions include tension, tremor, strategies to cope with the perseveration of disfluency (e.g., slowing down during the repetitions or sudden arrest of phonation), vocal fry, interrupter reactions or attempts to overcome the blocks, speaking on expiratory reserve, respiratory gasps (used to interrupt the closure of the airway), and speaking on inhalation. Reactions to the fear of stuttering, in contrast to reactions to the experience of stuttering, are motivated by internal states of mind and emotions that must be inferred from the overt symptoms. Although the manifestations of these reactions to the fear of stuttering are numerous, they are basically motivated by attempts to avoid, postpone, start, or disguise the stuttering.

Behaviors motivated by avoidance include attempted evasion of specific communication situations or words, substitutions or circumlocutions, and use of unusual ways of speaking such as speaking rapidly or with an unusual cadence. Postponement can take the form of silent intervals, certain facial or bodily movements, and use of interjections. Starters are the behaviors a stutterer uses in attempts to get himself started on a word, often after a period of postponement. Starters may involve intricate timing of verbal and nonverbal behaviors that range from repetitions of words already spoken normally to get a "running start" on the feared word, to head nods, to assuming a preparatory set of the articulators for an upcoming word. The preparatory set may or may not be appropriate to the upcoming syllable. Disguise reactions are motivated by attempts to hide or camouflage one's stuttering, including bodily movements, inappropriate laughter, or adopting another voice pattern.

Through successive failures at speaking fluently, according to Van Riper, the more advanced stutterer accrues certain overt and covert behaviors in an effort to reduce stuttering. Such behaviors may have been effective when first used, but their efficacy becomes diluted as the novelty of the response wears off. Yet the strength of the response is likely to increase because of intermittent reinforcement. These responses are symptomatic of the stutterer's affective reactions and his or her attempt to search for the proper timing needed for the complex coarticulatory movements of speech.

The covert, affective reactions to stuttering encompass the emotional aspects of stuttering, either in anticipation of speech failure or as a response to failure. Although some stutter without accompanying emotionality, foremost among the affective responses for the others are fear, anxiety, frustration, guilt, and hostility. These feelings can be specific to particular speaking situations, listeners, and topics of conversation. Increased propositionality or meaning and increased information load in a message often carry a greater probability for fluency breakdowns. According to Van Riper, stuttering is a disorder not only of speech but also of communication in that the receiver of the message can have a great impact on the stutterer. Although the covert reactions revolve around the stutterer's emotions and feelings, these emotions can have physiological correlates stemming from both the central and the autonomic nervous systems. Muscular tension, for example, may accompany moments of heightened emotion. The autonomic nervous system functions to maintain physiological homeostasis. That is, the sympathetic branch of the autonomic system is capable of providing certain "emergency" reactions such as an increase in the force of contraction of each heart beat and in the amount of light falling on the retina, an increase in the secretion of adrenaline, and faster and deeper breathing (Sternbach, 1966). On the other hand, the parasympathetic branch of the autonomic nervous system governs the initiation and maintenance of such processes as digestion and metabolism, as well as counteracting specific functions of the sympathetic branch, such as constriction of the pupil and slowing down of heart rate. Most organs in the body are supplied by nerves from both branches of the autonomic nervous system, which function together toward autonomic balance. Anxiety, according to Gellhorn (1965), occurs when the autonomic nervous system is "tuned" more toward sympathetic arousal.

Bloodstein (1981) places stuttering responses into two main categories: 1) the essential, integral, or primary features of stuttering, which include repetitions, prolongations, and pauses; and 2) the associated, secondary, or concomitant features of stuttering. The latter group of symptoms usually but not necessarily occurs immediately adjacent to or concurrent with the actual interruptions of speech associated with the primary features of stuttering. Moreover, Bloodstein views the associated symptoms as belonging to three categories: the overt, the physiological, and the introspective concomitants of stuttering. The overt concomitants include certain visible or audible behaviors such as associated movements (eye blinks, head jerks); interjected speech fragments (superfluous and at times inappropriate interjections); vocal anomalies (rapid or slow rate of speech, changes in vocal quality and pitch); and visible dermal reactions such as flushing or pallor. The physiological concomitants are the more covert, internal bodily changes due primarily to momentary heightening of emotional arousal. These physiological concomitants, similar to Van Riper's "covert reactions," include subtle eye movements, cardiovascular changes, tremors, EEG changes, biochemical disturbances, electrodermal disturbances, and other reflex activities such as pupil dilation. Bloodstein advises that these physiological concomitants are merely momentary reactions to specific instances of stuttering rather than chronic traits that bear etiological significance. The third group of associated symptoms, the introspective concomitants, consists of subjective evaluations that stutterers, typically older stutterers, offer to express their feelings related to stuttering. These introspections include feelings of frustration in not being able to get on with the speech act, feelings of muscular strain and tension, and emotional reactions that occur before, during, or after a block. Typically, feelings associated with the anticipation of a block include fear and anxiety; feelings associated with the block itself include a loss of perceptual contact with one's immediate surroundings; and feelings associated with moments following a block include frustration, embarrassment, guilt for some, and a possible reduction of tension and a sense of relief for others.

In Chapter 6, Table 2 (pp. 144–145) offers a matrix, based largely on Van Riper's schema, by which one can systematically assess the behavioral dimensions of stuttering. The matrix is organized around three major categories: general fluency and language information, the core behaviors of stuttering, and accompanying symptoms. The first category covers information about the size of the child's corpus from which the analysis was made, the mean length of utterance (MLU), if appropriate, and overall ratings of the child's speech rate, stuttering severity, and loci of stuttering. The second category summarizes information on the core or essential behaviors of stuttering, consisting of repetitions, prolongations, and tense pauses. The final category delineates behaviors resulting from reactions to the core behaviors and from reactions to the fear of stuttering. For a more detailed discussion of the matrix, refer to Chapter 6.

CHARACTERISTICS OF CHILDREN WHO STUTTER

Characteristics in Relation to Selected Issues

Normal Nonfluencies versus Pathological Disfluencies   At the core of the issue of normal nonfluencies versus abnormal disfluencies is the validity of the continuity hypothesis, which asserts that there is continuity between the mild fragmentations of speech characteristic of normal youngsters and the speech disruptions characteristic of young stutterers. Researchers and clinicians have had to delineate what they considered to be the normally nonfluent from the abnormally disfluent youngsters as they conducted research and differential diagnosis. Differentiating the two types of speech may be difficult at the very earliest onset of stuttering because of great individual variations and because even such traits as sound prolongation and tense pauses characterize the speech of some normally speaking 2-year-olds (Yairi, 1981). Moreover, in some of the classic work on early stuttering, such as the Iowa Studies, the diagnoses were based in part on long-term recollections by parents.

Some representative studies attempting to differentiate normal from abnormal fluency patterns during childhood are summarized next, beginning with the Iowa Studies.

The Iowa Studies The Iowa Studies by Johnson and Associates (1959) summarized data on a series of comparisons of children who stuttered with those who did not. Part of the data was based on parental interviews and part consisted of comparing the two groups (ages 2.5 to 8 years) in terms of eight categories of disfluencies. The eight categories were: interjections, sound and syllable repetitions, word repetitions, phrase repetitions, revisions (e.g., "I was—I am going"), incomplete phrases (e.g., "I was—and after she got there, he came"), broken words (e.g., "I was g-(pause)-oing home"), and prolonged sounds. Analyses indicated that the group frequency index means for the categories of sound, syllable, word and phrase repetitions, and sound prolongations most distinguished the stutterers from the controls for the male subjects, followed by broken words. Interjections, revisions, and incomplete phrases did not differentiate the two groups of male children.

For the girls, sound, syllable, and word repetitions differentiated the two groups most, followed by prolonged sounds. Mean differences were not significant for the interjections, phrase repetitions, revisions, incomplete phrases, and broken words (Johnson and Associates, 1959). Moreover, stutterers showed a greater mean number of units per repetition (e.g., *su-, su-, su-, sun* has three units of repetitions) than did the normal youngsters. Johnson also pointed to the overlapping between the two groups of children, in that all eight of the disfluency categories were shared to some degree by both groups of children. The findings of this study and of the related investigations referred to suggest that most, and possibly all, very young children speak with sufficient nonfluency to be classified as "stutterers" by appropriately motivated parents or by other listeners (Johnson and Associates, 1959). Johnson used this interpretation of the data to reaffirm his diagnosogenic theory of childhood stuttering.

McDearmon (1968) reexamined some of the data from Johnson's study and added some more detailed perspectives on the early nonfluency patterns of children. His conclusions included the following:

> *This study indicates that controls and experimentals at onset were strongly differentiated, not only in the incidence of specific nonfluency reactions that Johnson (1959, p. 135) found, but in the incidence of tension, "normal nonfluency," and "primary stuttering." It tends to confirm Van Riper's (1963, p. 328) description of primary stuttering, which specified repetitions and prolongations of sounds and syllables, not pauses or repetitions of words and phrases. . . . The results of this study tend to support Bloodstein's (1958, pp. 15–34) findings of overlapping and lack of sharp distinction between primary and secondary stuttering. . . . At the same time, these results, while tending to confirm Johnson's findings of overlapping between primary stuttering and normal nonfluency, do not support his rejection of the general distinction between these two behaviors either*
> (McDearmon, 1968, p. 636).

Other Studies   In one of the earliest works tracing the fluency characteristics of young children, Davis (1939) found that most of normal children's repetitions consisted of word and phrase repetitions. Van Riper, in the third edition of *Speech Correction: Principles and Method* (1954) cited sound and syllable repetitions as characteristic of stutterers whereas word and phrase repetitions are common to both normals and stutterers.

In an interesting study to see whether an interaction exists between quantitative increases in disfluencies versus qualitative changes, Yairi (1972) compared the proportion of disfluency types to the total number of disfluencies of low and highly disfluent nonstutterers and the same for stutterers. Subjects' ages averaged 8 years 9 months. Yairi found that the disfluency types were proportionally similar for the two subgroups of nonstutterers. However, an interaction effect existed between quantitative and qualitative changes for the young stutterers. In particular, the more disfluent stutterers showed increases in the proportion of interjections, part-word repetitions, whole-word repetitions, disrhythmic phonation, and tense pauses, but decreases in the proportion of revisions and phrase repetitions. Congruent with others' findings, such as Van Riper's cited above, part-word repetitions seem to carry great distinction in that the proportion of part-word repetitions was small relative to the total disfluencies for the nonstuttering children but was high for the stuttering group.

Motivated by the rationale that incipient stutterers are less facile in coordinating movements required for fluent speech, Floyd and Perkins (1974) reasoned that young stutterers should exhibit a high rate of syllable breakdowns. The investigators examined the fluency behaviors of 4 stutterers and 20 nonstutterers 3 to 5 years of age during free play with their mothers. Results indicated that the stuttering group had a mean of 9.88% syllables disfluent, whereas the nonstuttering group showed a mean of 1.24% syllables disfluent. Floyd and Perkins speculated that incipient young stutterers may be less able to manage the coordination necessary for fluency from the start.

Bjerkan (1980) compared 108 normal preschoolers with 2 young stutterers. A major demarcation between the two sets of children is that word fragmentations most distinguished the stutterers. Such word fragmentations include part-word repetitions, sound prolongations, blockings, and interjections within a word. Syllable repetitions were also quite prevalent in the early stuttering observed by parents of 2- and 3-year-old children studied by Yairi (1983). Moreover, the number of repetition units may have potential diagnostic significance.

Age of the Child Stutterer   The age of the young stutterer has been a major parameter in differentiating symptoms as well as in determining the therapeutic approaches to childhood stuttering. Clinicians have traditionally treated the disfluent preschooler differently from the older disfluent child. The various developmental stages and phases detailed later in this chapter also project the generalization that as the child gets older, likewise the pattern of his stuttering progresses from one stage or phase to the next. Although the latter has intuitive appeal and may be a valid generalization for a fair portion of youngsters, Wingate (1976) rightfully points to exceptions. In particular, Wingate notes that some stutterers plateau in the severity of their stuttering, whereas a good number of others show spontaneous remission.

The seminal work on loci of stuttering by Brown (1937), on adults, served to focus attention in later studies on the relation between grammatical functions and disfluency for children of different ages. "Grammatical function" in the Brown study referred to the finding that adult stutterers stuttered with significantly higher frequency on parts of speech that are nouns, verbs, adjectives, and adverbs than on articles, prepositions, pronouns, and conjunctions.

Bloodstein (1981) has been instrumental in pointing out some intrinsic and significant differences in the fluency patterns of children as a function of age. In a study of 13 preschool stutterers, for example, Bloodstein and Gantwerk (1967) examined the influence of the grammatical function of words on the distribution of stuttering during free play. Results did not yield the same grammatical factor influencing stuttering patterns as in adults because most disfluencies were randomly distributed with respect to parts of speech. However, the rate of occurrence of stuttering on pronouns and conjunctions tended to be greater than chance expectation. Upon closer examination, the authors concluded that there is a strong "positional effect" of these two classes of words because they occur frequently at the beginning of phrases.

In a similar study but with 15 normally fluent preschoolers, Helmreich and Bloodstein (1973) compared the percentage of the children's nonfluent words with the percentage of their total words, which fell into various grammatical categories. Results were similar to the findings by Bloodstein and Gantwerk (1967) in that there was a preponderance of fluency disruptions on pronouns and conjunctions at the beginning of utterances. The data were used to support the continuity hypothesis. A study by Williams, Silverman, and Kools (1969) exemplifies the contention that patterns of disfluencies for the older child stutterer become more adultlike with age. In particular, Williams et al. found more salient word-bound effects for the 5- to 13-year-old stutterers and normals they studied; that is, greater disfluencies occurred on verbs, nouns, adverbs, and adjectives.

Bloodstein (1981, pp. 288–289, 317) cited the following stimuli on which older children stutter to support the notion that the stuttering of older children (and adults) is more word bound than that of preschool stutterers: content words, words beginning with consonants, longer words, and words carrying greater information load (i.e., less predictability of occurrence).

Individual Variations of Symptomatology   Investigators in the field of communication disorders are becoming increasingly aware of the importance of individual differences, ranges of normality, and the existence of subgroups of individuals within a particular pathology. Such heterogeneity can have profound implications for the assessment and treatment of childhood stuttering, as well as for research. The model around which our assessment and treatment approaches are organized consists of three interlocking factors: the psychosocial, physiological, and psycholinguistic factors. One quickly allows room for individual variations of symptomatology when one realizes the complex dynamics of the individual variables under each factor for any given child. Peer influence under the psychosocial factor, for example, will differ across children as a function of the kinds of peer reaction a young stutterer perceives, as well as the interpretation of such perceptions by that child. Variations in learning histories of the stuttering responses, which seem to span all three factors, can also contribute to individual differences in symptomatology and, in turn, treatment approaches.

Subtypes of Stutterers   Related to individual variations of symptomatology is the issue of subtypes of stutterers. Subtypes arise from intrinsic differences between clusters of stutterers, due to either etiological or symptomatological differences. Most categories of fluency disorders discussed in the literature have been developed through clinical observation. Data based on empirical research to verify the existence of these subtypes remain scarce. However, Conture and his associates at Syracuse University are currently attempting to develop clusters of child stutterers based on various analyses of behaviors (Caruso, Schwartz, and Conture, 1983; Conture and Schwartz, 1984; Schwartz, dissertation in progress, Syracuse University).

Andrews and Harris (1964) arrived at certain factors that may contribute to stuttering. These factors include heredity, poor speech development, and an overall "lack of capacity to think, talk and behave" (p. 117).

It is of interest to note that another group of clients with fluency anomalies, namely the clutterers, also experience deficits in thinking and speaking/language skills. Clutterers are said to have a "central language imbalance," whereby difficulties in speech, language, and fluency coexist. Some authors accentuate similarities in symptoms between the clutterer and the stutterer, whereas others accentuate the differences between these two groups (Luchsinger and Arnold, 1965; Myers, 1982). According to Weiss (1964), for example, stuttering and cluttering are rather closely aligned. Weiss speculates that the two pathologies lie on a continuum, and that stuttering evolves from cluttering during very early childhood. Although stuttering and cluttering in their respective "pure" states can be differentiated in terms of some of the symptoms (e.g., generally faster overall rate for clutterers compared to stutterers), both cluttering and stuttering behaviors can coexist in the same individual.

Cluttering-stuttering, a "specifically inherited and organically caused" problem, represents only one of the six subtypes of stutterer outlined by Luchsinger and Arnold (1965). The second subtype comprises symptomatic stutterers whose condition is due to lesions of brain function, such as rate disturbances following birth injury, encephalitis, or head trauma. The third subgroup consists of children with developmental stuttering attributable to "familial psychoneurotic tendencies." The role of imitation and certain psychological explanations of stuttering are also pertinent to the third subgroup. The fourth type of stuttering is physiological stuttering, and best supports Johnson's diagnosogenic theory in that the normal nonfluencies of childhood are exacerbated into physiological stuttering by adverse reactions from adults to the child's speech. The fifth and sixth categories are, respectively, traumatic stuttering resulting from immense stress, and hysterical stuttering due to conversion reaction in individuals suffering from "constitutional psychopathy."

Besides the four tracks or subgroups of childhood stutterers discussed in detail under "The Development of Stuttering" later in this chapter, Van Riper describes tonic versus clonic stuttering, and interiorized versus exteriorized stutterers. Tonic stuttering is characterized by the relatively sustained contraction of the speech musculatures, which contributes to the "fixatory" behaviors of disfluencies. Clonic stuttering is characterized by repetitive or oscillatory motion during speech, resulting in such behaviors as syllable or sound repetitions. Van Riper cautions that these two types of stuttering behavior overlap a great deal and, in fact, are not usually clearly delineated.

Douglass and Quarrington (1952) differentiated types of stutterers on the basis of the relative prominence of their stuttering behaviors. The interiorized stutterer is covert about his disorder, exercising continual vigilance or avoidance, and consequently seems to be rather introverted. By contrast, the exteriorized stutterer is more open about his stuttering symptomatology. Van Riper views these two types of stuttering as different ways of reacting to the same basic disorder; he attributes them to different personality patterns or to different learning histories, rather than considering them to represent two intrinsically different types of stutterers.

Characteristics in Relation to Case History Information

This section is organized according to the psychosocial, physiological, and psycholinguistic factors, and their relevance to the symptoms of the young stutterer. The issues just discussed serve as a context for the present consideration of specific characteristics of children who stutter.

The Psychosocial Factor   The focal points of the psychosocial factor consist of important adults and peers in the child's life and, of course, the child's own psychosocial dynamics. Although a major theory of stuttering holds that stuttering emanates from neurosis and psychodynamic conflicts (e.g., Coriat, 1943; Barbara, 1954), by and large the research literature has not been able to verify that stutterers are any more or any less neurotic than the general population (Sheehan, 1958). Stutterers, as is the case with any other group of individuals, span the spectrum of personality types. Sheehan in 1970 reiterated that the concept of a single personality type governing stutterers is fallacious. In speaking of personality differences, one must be mindful of the difference between neuroticism as a personality type and bits of neurotic-like behaviors associated with the anticipation of moments of stuttering.

Because parents are the child's primary psychosocial agents during the early years of life, the impact of their influence is unquestioned. However, clinicians must not conclude that parents are a main factor influencing the onset and maintenance of stuttering children. Johnson's diagnosogenic theory of stuttering, having gained and sustained momentum in the field, may have aroused inadvertently a degree of guilt in the parents of young stutterers.

The research on parental attitudes and influences has yielded mixed results. The literature (e.g., Bloodstein, 1981, pp. 108–111) has alluded to different parenting styles as a function of differences in socioeconomic levels. The parents interviewed by Andrews and Harris (1964), for example, were of lower socioeconomic level than the parents interviewed by Johnson and his associates (1959). As in our discussion about the influences of personality, rather than looking at parental "types" per se, we should observe how parents and the young child interact in specific situations, particularly those that produce heightened disfluency. Borrowing from a hypothesis Johnson later set forth, stuttering must be evaluated in terms of the amount of disfluency in the child's speech, the parents' sensitivity to such disfluencies, and the child's reactions to his own speech and his sensitivity to the parents' reactions to his speech.

Some studies suggest that there may be a difference in parent-child dynamics of families of young stutterers. For example, Fowlie and Cooper (1978) studied traits attributed by mothers of 34 stuttering and 34 nonstuttering children using the Woods and Williams Adjective Checklist. They found that mothers of the stutterers perceived their children as being more sensitive, introverted, and anxious than did the mothers of the nonstuttering children. Moncur (1952) found that parents of stutterers tended to be more critical and domineering of their children than parents of nonstutterers.

In an interesting study analyzing utterances between parents and children, Kaprisin-Burrelli, Egolf, and Shames (1972) found that the parents of nonstuttering children gave more positive statements, and offered encouragement and understanding. Parents of the young stutterers, on the other hand, gave more negative reactions, such as interruptions, demands, and criticisms. Andrews and Harris (1964) compared mothers of stutterers and nonstutterers but did not find significant differences between the two groups on the Cattell Sixteen Personality Factor Inventory.

The Physiological Factor   With the possible exceptions of genetic predisposition and laryngeal/supralaryngeal differences, the literature has not been able to capture significant patterns of physiological deviancies that earmark stutterers as a group. Berry (1938) studied the medical case histories of numerous stutterers and their controls but found no significant differences between the two groups. The Newcastle studies by Andrews and Harris (1964) also did not find significant differences in, for example, incidence of diseases between eight stuttering children and their controls.

A major exception to the lack of significant difference between stutterers and nonstutterers is the possibility of a genetic predisposition to fluency breakdowns in some children. Clinical observations point to the prevalence of stuttering in families. Andrews and Harris speculated that stutterers, particularly female stutterers, have greater probabilities of having relatives who also stutter as a result of sex-linked genetic transmission of factors predisposing one toward stuttering. Van Riper (1982) also cites the higher incidence of stuttering in twins as opposed to nontwin siblings. One must be cautious, however, in deciding whether such data result exclusively from a genetic inheritance of factors predisposing one to stutter or whether one can also "inherit" certain familial sociological patterns that may be conducive to stuttering for some children.

The connection between intelligence and disfluency is equivocal. According to Bloodstein (1981), stutterers as a general rule are not any brighter or duller than nonstutterers. In their state-of-the-art review of the literature, on the other hand, Andrews et al. (1983) reported that school-aged stutterers score significantly (by 0.5 standard deviation) lower on intelligence tests than nonstutterers. Bloodstein suggests a possible subtle interaction effect between intelligence and socioeconomic level; that is, ". . . when surveys are extended to include low as well as high socioeconomic segments of the population, the mean IQ of stutterers may be slightly below the general average" (Bloodstein, 1981, p. 212).

The more microscopic types of physiological characteristics (i.e., those that are not easily or routinely uncovered in a case history), such as laryngeal musculature functioning or the coordination of the speech production system, are discussed in Chapter 5.

In reflecting on the significance and implications of the physiological data cited in the literature, we note first that as with the psychosocial and psycholinguistic factors, one must give due respect to the presence of individual differences. Second, conflicting or inconclusive results may simply reflect the state of the art. Our research paradigms need to be sharpened. The increased sophistication of the technological hardware that speech scientists can use gives hope of a more exacting scientific and ultimately a more enlightened clinical approach to the assessment and treatment of childhood stuttering.

The Psycholinguistic Factor   Momentum has been gained in the past decade on the study of the possible relations between language and fluency development during early childhood. Language, perhaps even more than the production of speech sounds, is at the heart of communication development during the early preschool years. Language development represents the culmination of development in such other critical areas as cognition and socialization. These areas are intrinsically intermeshed. In perusing a child's case history, therefore, one must consider his or her linguistic skills in the context of the cognitive and psychosocial underpinnings of communication.

Chapter 4 provides an in-depth review and discussion of the psycholinguistic aspects of childhood stuttering. This section highlights some generalizations on the psycholinguistic aspects of fluency development that may bear on the examination of the case history of a young disfluent child.

The literature points to a distinct possibility of some language delay in some young stutterers or even in some normal but nonetheless highly disfluent children (Muma, 1971). The nature of this relationship is yet to be mapped out. Nonetheless, age seems to be a key variable in determining the distribution of disfluencies in a child's language output. In particular, older children tend to be more disfluent on words that begin with consonants, are members of the content word class, and are relatively longer (Bloodstein, 1981). Preschoolers tend to stutter at the beginning of syntactic units (Bloodstein, 1974; Wall, Starkweather, and Cairns, 1981). Because conjunctions and pronouns have a high rate of occurrence at the beginning of utterances, Bloodstein and Gantwerk (1967) found that although the disfluencies of young stutterers occurred on all parts of speech, they were particularly evident on pronouns and conjunctions.

It is difficult to separate syntax, semantics, and pragmatics during natural discourse; nevertheless, a child may experience relative strengths and weaknesses in one of these areas of language compared to the others. Semantics has been considered in general terms as the study of meaning, but it can also carry specific notions such as the propositionality of an utterance (Eisenson, 1975), or the development of semantic-syntactic structures (Colburn and Mysak, 1982a, 1982b). A proposition, according to Eisenson, is an "intellectually meaningful linguistic unit." Utterances carrying greater propositionality often incur greater amounts of stuttering because of the meaningfulness of the utterance in the particular pragmatic context. Utterances spoken in situations that carry greater communicative intent or stress often trigger greater amounts of disfluencies, both for normal youngsters and stutterers (e.g., Davis, 1939, 1940a, 1940b).

THE DEVELOPMENT OF STUTTERING

Ideally, developmental trends of childhood stuttering should be based on longitudinal studies whereby the same group of children are traced throughout their respective developmental progressions. Such studies are rare because so much time and effort are needed to collect data over the span of years. Several authors have offered schemas to trace the developmental trends of childhood stuttering. Few meet the mark of a rigorous longitudinal study, given the inherent difficulties of such a study. Nonetheless, the schemas that are offered are based on years of clinical albeit cross-sectional research experience.

Bluemel, Froeschels, Van Riper, and Bloodstein

Bluemel (1932) was one of the first to coin the terms "primary" and "secondary stammering." Primary stammering or stuttering is characterized by the easy and effortless repetitions of syllables and words at the beginning of an utterance, with little or no awareness by the child but with great episodicity; the fluency disruptions come and go, wax and wane. Secondary stuttering emerges when the disfluencies become more effortful and persistent. The child is more aware if not more anxious about the stuttering and, in time, begins to use specific devices (such as starters) to reduce the blocks. Bluemel viewed stuttering as a habit learned through conditioning. Part of the conditioning is instigated by the adverse stimuli and responses from others, so that in time young stutterers also "learn" that they have difficulty with speech. Such perceptions of speech difficulty in turn lead to further struggle and fear, thereby worsening the stuttering.

Froeschels (1964) viewed the onset and development of stuttering as a progression whereby the initially effortless repetitions using normal speech rate gradually accrue greater tension, first with a faster rate of speech and later with a slower rate of speech as the child struggles with words. Froeschels was one of the first to distinguish tonic from clonic types of stuttering (viz., the sustained, hard types of block and the repetitive or oscillatory types of block, respectively). He added that "concealed stuttering" represents a very advanced form or stage of stuttering whereby individuals develop strategies to hide their stuttering. Douglass and Quarrington (1952) distinguished the interiorized from the exteriorized stutterer. The interiorized stutterer, similar to Froeschel's notion of the "concealed stuttering," is one who attempts to hide the overt symptoms of his stuttering.

Van Riper's earlier thinking (1954, 1963) about the development of stuttering expanded on Bluemel's notion of a primary and a secondary stage of stuttering. Van Riper added some transitional characteristics to include changes in speech rate and an increase in awareness of and, later, emotional reactions to the fluency disruptions. In 1982, however, Van Riper further refined his ideas about the development of stuttering: not only are there developmental stages for any given child, but also there are developmental stages associated with different subgroups of young stutterers. Such insights regarding the heterogeneity of childhood stuttering boosted our appreciation of the complexity of developmental stuttering tremendously. Based on an examination of 300 case histories of child stutterers Van Riper and his associates had seen, including 44 case histories and clinical records with sufficient longitudinal data, Van Riper distilled four tracks of development.

Track I, comprising the greatest percentage of young stutterers, is marked by a gradual onset of disfluencies after a period of fluency. Onset usually occurs around 2.5 to 4 years of age, and the disfluencies are quite oscillatory in the beginning, consisting primarily of syllable repetitions with very little tension or awareness. The pacing of these syllable repetitions becomes more irregular, and the events become more frequent in time. Furthermore, the child begins to exhibit more and more sound prolongations. Tension, frustration, fear, and avoidance are the earmarks of the later stages of the Track I child.

Track II, also representing a relatively large group of children, is marked by an onset that is concurrent with the very beginnings of speech and language development, so that the child has never been very fluent from the start. The Track II child is of particular interest to language pathologists because he or she can also have concomitant articulation and language difficulties. Although there is little or no tension or awareness at the beginning, the child's awareness develops gradually and the rate of speech quickens. Some of the attributes of Track II overlap with traits characterizing a young clutterer.

Tracks III and IV are relatively less common. The onset of the third track is marked by the sudden initiation of stuttering in a previously fluent child, often after a traumatic event. From the beginning, the child experiences great tension, with symptoms of laryngeal blockings, unvoiced prolongations, and slow and deliberate rate of speech. The child is highly aware of the disfluencies from the onset, and experiences frustration and situation- and word-specific fears. Progression of the Track III child is rather rapid and morbid, characterized by hard blocks, struggles, body and limb movements, and increased frustration. This progression culminates in intense fears resulting in avoidances, very severe stuttering, and perhaps even signs of interiorized stuttering.

The hallmark of the Track IV stutterer is the rather stylized and contrived disfluencies. Onset is sudden, usually after the child has been fluent. Such children are highly aware of their stuttering but show no sign of frustration or fear. In fact, they show little affect toward their stuttering, which at times seems to be stereotypic and deliberate. It is as if they were "offering" the stuttering to the listener. Little change in the disfluency patterns occurs except for increases in the duration and visibility of the stuttering. The Track IV child continues to show little avoidance or fear, although quite aware of the stuttering. He or she continues to be very verbal and stutters openly, unlike the Track III child who becomes more and more introverted.

Bloodstein (1981) offers a four-phase schema to describe the development of stuttering in children. His precautionary notes about not universally generalizing the phases nor assuming that any given child will abruptly enter from one phase to the next are well taken. Bloodstein's Phase 1 is marked by great episodicity, prevalence of whole-word repetitions (especially at the beginning of sentences, clauses, or phrases), and relatively little concern about one's disfluencies. The disfluencies become more chronic during Phase 2, and the child begins to identify himself as a stutterer although he remains relatively unconcerned. The child is especially disfluent under conditions of heightened excitement or when speaking very rapidly.

Phase 3 is distinguished by inhibitions that are specific to speaking situations, words, or sounds. Word substitutions and circumlocutions develop. Finally, during the fourth stage, the stutterer has accrued a great deal of fear and anticipation and, in turn, tends to avoid speaking situations. Although Phase 4 is most often associated with later adolescence or adulthood, Bloodstein indicates that the symptoms may also prevail during late childhood. The stutterer becomes quite sensitive to his stuttering, to the point that interpersonal interactions with others may be impaired.

Critique of a "Stages" or "Phases" Approach to the Study of Developmental Stuttering

Although the foregoing schemas for the development of stuttering have undoubtedly been helpful to clinicians in projecting a general outline for the progression of stuttering, adhering strictly to a "stages" approach may impose limitations.

Wingate (1976, pp. 63–67) reviews two lines of criticism of a "stages" approach. The first rests on the validity of a continuity hypothesis, under which a distinction between normal nonfluencies and the disfluencies of early "primary" stuttering is not justifiable. Moreover, using a special term such as "primary" stuttering may generate in the child negative reactions to his own speech. Wingate, however, maintains that a distinction can be inferred between normal nonfluencies and incipient stuttering, based on the data presented earlier in his book *Stuttering: Theory and Treatment* (1976). Therefore, the first line of criticism "has no credibility, and hence . . . no substance" (Wingate, 1976, p. 63).

The second line of criticism, which Wingate espouses, rests on the notion that symptoms of the primary stage of stuttering are not necessarily distinguishable from symptoms of the secondary stage. A critical feature of the secondary stage is awareness of stuttering and effortfulness during the speech act, according to Bluemel and his followers. Determination of awareness in a child, however, is usually arrived at through subjective judgment and inference.

Implicit if not explicit in a "stages" approach to the study of developmental stuttering is the tenet that stuttering, particularly in children who have not been treated, becomes progressively worse. This tenet has, unfortunately, been verified in a good many of our clinical cases. However, holding strictly to a "stages" approach excludes other possibilities: 1) that the symptoms remain unchanged, 2) that the symptoms show great periodicity and fluctuations, 3) that the symptoms remit spontaneously, 4) that stuttering is severe even at onset during early childhood, and 5) that the stuttering of older clients is very mild. In summary, ". . . we have absolutely no grounds for predicting either course or destination for any case of stuttering" (Wingate, 1976, p. 67). Wingate advocates terms such as "simple" or "complicated" behaviors of stuttering.

Bloodstein (1981) offers his developmental sequence of stuttering with some precautionary notes about a "stages" approach. In particular, Bloodstein notes the following qualifications: 1) some early childhood stutterers experience heightened although transient emotional reactions to their disfluencies, 2) the presence of secondary symptoms does not necessarily mean that a child is pervasively fearful of speaking, and 3) childhood stuttering is not dichotomous but is continuous both with normal childhood nonfluencies and between the so-called primary and secondary stages of stuttering.

Van Riper also cautions clinicians about developmental schemas based solely on cross-sectional data, such as information obtained from an initial interview with parents. His developmental trends, however, are strengthened by the delineation of possible subgroups of young stutterers as well as by basing part of the descriptions of the four tracks on longitudinal data.

REFERENCES

Andrews, G., Craig, A., Feyer, A.-M., Hoddinott, S., Howie, P., and Neilson, M. 1983. Stuttering: A review of research findings circa 1982. J. Speech Hear. Disord. 48:226–246.

Andrews, G., and Harris, M. 1964. The Syndrome of Stuttering. Clinics in Developmental Medicine, no. 17. Spastics Society Medical, Education and Information Unit in association with William Heinemann Medical Books, London.

Barbara, D. 1954. Stuttering: A Psychodynamic Approach to Its Understanding and Treatment. Julian Press, New York.

Berry, M. 1938. Developmental history of stuttering children. J. Pediatr. 12:209–217.

Bjerkan, B. 1980. Word fragmentations and repetitions in the spontaneous speech of 2–6-year-old children. J. Fluency Disord. 5:137–148.

Bloodstein, O. 1958. Stuttering as an anticipatory struggle reaction. In: J. Eisenson (ed.), Stuttering: A Symposium. pp. 1–69. Harper & Row, New York.

Bloodstein, O. 1974. The rules of early stuttering. J. Speech Hear. Disord. 39:379–394.

Bloodstein, O. 1981. A Handbook on Stuttering. 3rd Ed. National Easter Seal Society, Chicago.

Bloodstein, O., and Gantwerk, B. 1967. Grammatical function in relation to stuttering in young children. J. Speech Hear. Res. 10:786–789.

Bluemel, C, 1932. Primary and secondary stammering. Q. J. Speech. 18:187–200.

Brady, W., and Hall, D. 1976. The prevalence of stuttering among school-age children. Lang. Speech Hear. Serv. Schools. 7:75–81.

Brown, S. 1937. The influence of grammatical function on the incidence of stuttering. J. Speech Disord. 2:207–215.

Canter, G. 1971. Observations on neurogenic stuttering: A contribution to differential diagnosis. Br. J. Disord. Commun. 6:139–143.

Caruso, A., Schwartz, H. D., and Conture, E. 1983. Children who stutter: A behavioral/physiological perspective. Short course presented at the National Conference of the American Speech-Language-Hearing Association, Cincinnati.

Colburn, N., and Mysak, E. 1982a. Developmental disfluency and emerging grammar. 1. Disfluency characteristics in early syntactic utterances. J. Speech Hear. Res. 25:414–420.

Colburn, N., and Mysak, E. 1982b. Developmental disfluency and emerging grammar. II. Co-occurrence of disfluency with specified semantic-syntactic structures. J. Speech Hear. Res. 25:421–427.

Conture, E., and Schwartz, H. D. 1984. Children who stutter: Diagnosis and remediation. Commun. Disord. 9:1–18.

Cooper, E., Parris, R., and Wells, M. 1974. Prevalence of the recovery from speech disorders in a group of freshmen at the University of Alabama. A.S.H.A. 16(abstr.):359–360.

Coriat, I. 1943. The psychoanalytic concept of stammering. Nerv. Child. 2:167–171.

Davis, D. 1939. The relation of repetitions in the speech of young children to certain measures of language maturity and situational factors: Part I. J. Speech Disord. 4:303–318.

Davis, D. 1940a. The relation of repetitions in the speech of young children to certain measures of language maturity and situational factors: Part II. J. Speech Disord. 5:235–241.

Davis, D. 1940b. The relation of repetitions in the speech of young children to certain measures of language maturity and situational factors: Part III. J. Speech Disord. 5:242–246.

DeJoy, D., and Gregory, H. 1975. The developmental nature of fluency in children: Data from two preschool age groups. Paper presented at the National Conference of the American Speech-Language-Hearing Association, Washington, D.C.

Dickson, S. 1971. Incipient stuttering and spontaneous remission of stuttered speech. J. Commun. Disord. 4:99–110.

Douglass, E., and Quarrington, B. 1952. The differentiation of interiorized and exteriorized secondary stuttering. J. Speech Hear. Disord. 17:377–385.

Eisenson, J. 1975. Stuttering as perseverative behavior. In: J. Eisenson (ed.), Stuttering: A Second Symposium, pp. 401–452. Harper & Row, New York.

Floyd, S., and Perkins, W. 1974. Early syllable dysfluency in stutterers and nonstutterers: A preliminary report. J. Commun. Disord. 7:279–282.

Fowlie, G., and Cooper, E. 1978. Traits attributed to stuttering and nonstuttering children by their mothers. J. Fluency Disord. 3:233–246.

Froeschels, E. 1964. Selected Papers (1940–1964). North-Holland, Amsterdam.

Gellhorn, E. 1965. The neurophysiological basis of anxiety: A hypothesis. Perspect. Biol. Med. 8:488–515.

Gillespie, S., and Cooper, E. 1973. Prevalence of speech problems in junior and senior high schools. J. Speech Hear. Res. 16:739–743.

Glasner, P., and Rosenthal, D. 1957. Parental diagnosis of stuttering in young children. J. Speech Hear. Disord. 22:288–295.

Helm, N., Butler, R., and Canter, G. 1980. Neurogenic acquired stuttering. J. Fluency Disord. 5:269–279.

Helmreich, H., and Bloodstein, O. 1973. The grammatical factor in childhood disfluency in relation to the continuity hypothesis. J. Speech Hear. Res. 16:731–738.

Henderson, A., Goldman-Eisler, F., and Skarbek, A. 1966. Sequential temporal patterns in spontaneous speech. Lang. Speech. 9:207–216.

Johnson, W., and Associates. 1959. The Onset of Stuttering. University of Minnesota Press, Minneapolis.

Kaprisin-Burrelli, A., Egolf, D., and Shames, G. 1972. A comparison of parental verbal behavior with stuttering and nonstuttering children. J. Commun. Disord. 5:335–346.

Kidd, K., Kidd, J., and Records, M. 1978. The possible causes of the sex ratio in stuttering and its implications. J. Fluency Disord. 3:13–23.

Luchsinger, R., and Arnold, G. 1965. Voice-Speech-Language, Clinical Communicology: Its Physiology. Wadsworth Publishing Company, Belmont, Calif.

McDearmon, J. 1968. Primary stuttering at the onset of stuttering: A re-examination of data. J. Speech Hear. Res. 11:631–637.

Moncur, J. 1952. Parental domination in stuttering. J. Speech Hear. Disord. 17:155–165.

Muma, J. 1971. Syntax of preschool fluent and disfluent speech: A transformational analysis. J. Speech Hear. Res. 14:428–441.

Myers, F. 1982. Acoustic and perceptual characteristics of cluttering. Paper presented at the 22nd New York State Speech-Language-Hearing Association Convention, April 25–28, Ellenville, N.Y.

Sheehan, J. 1958. Conflict theory of stuttering. In: J. Eisenson (ed.), Stuttering: A Symposium, pp. 121–166. Harper & Row, New York.

Sheehan, J. 1970. Stuttering: Research and Therapy. Harper & Row, New York.

Starkweather, C. 1980. Speech fluency and its development in normal children. In: N. Lass (ed.), Speech and Language: Advances in Basic Research and Practice, pp. 143–200, Vol. 4. Academic Press, New York.

Sternbach, R. 1966. Principles of Psychophysiology. Academic Press, New York.

Van Riper, C. 1954. Speech Correction: Principles and Methods. 3rd Ed. Prentice-Hall, Englewood Cliffs, N.J.

Van Riper, C. 1963. Speech Correction: Principles and Methods. 4th Ed. Prentice-Hall, Englewood Cliffs, N.J.

Van Riper, C. 1982. The Nature of Stuttering. 2nd Ed. Prentice-Hall, Englewood Cliffs, N.J.

Wall, M., Starkweather, C., and Cairns, H. 1981. Syntactic influences on stuttering in young child stutterers. J. Fluency Disord. 6:283–298.

Weiss, D. 1964. Cluttering. Prentice-Hall, Englewood Cliffs, N.J.

Williams, D., Silverman, F., and Kools, J. 1969. Disfluency behavior of elementary-school stutterers and nonstutterers: Loci of instances of disfluency. J. Speech Hear. Res. 12:308–318.

Wingate, M. 1964. A standard definition of stuttering. J. Speech Hearing Disord. 29:484–489.

Wingate, M. 1976. Stuttering: Theory and Treatment. John Wiley & Sons, New York.

Yairi, E. 1972. Disfluency rates and patterns of stutterers and nonstutterers. J. Commun. Disord. 5:225–231.

Yairi, E. 1981. Disfluencies of normally speaking two-year-old children. J. Speech Hearing Res. 24:490–495.

Yairi, E. 1983. The onset of stuttering in two- and three-year-old children: A preliminary report. J. Speech Hear. Disord. 48:171–177.

4
Psycholinguistic Aspects of Childhood Stuttering

HISTORICAL PERSPECTIVE ON THE STUDY OF DEVELOPMENTAL PSYCHOLINGUISTICS

Although clinicians have always been interested in the speech and language development of children, the theory of child language and the practice of language therapy have not always been clearly delineated or well tuned. The field of child language has made great strides since the 1950s and 1960s. Indeed, a historical perspective would be helpful to understand the current trends in the study of child language and the treatment of its disorders, and how these recent trends may enlighten us on the relation between language and fluency in particular.

The Pre-Chomsky Era

Speech pathologists concerned with children's speech and language development during the 1950's and early 1960's were primarily interested in the development of articulatory skills, the growth of vocabulary, and selected aspects of children's linguistic structures. Besides the use of tests such as the Peabody Picture Vocabulary Test (PPVT (Dunn, 1965, Rev. Ed., 1981)), speech correctionists also analyzed speech samples using such measures as mean length of response (McCarthy, 1954) and structural complexity indices (Templin, 1957). The latter included an examination of completeness of response and occurrences of simple compared to complex or compound sentences.

Chomsky and Skinner

Noam Chomsky and B. F. Skinner are indeed strange bedfellows. Their approaches to language are diametrically opposite. The two, however, imposed a profound impact on the field at about the same time. Skinner, the psychologist, espoused a behavioral approach to learning, in which most if not all behaviors are seen to be learned through a stimulus-response paradigm. When both stimuli for and consequences of behavior, including language, are appropriately programmed, the desired bit of behavior presumably increases. Skinner gave little if any concern to the affective or cognitive aspects of behavior, except in discussions of respondent conditioning. Chomsky reviewed Skinner's approach to verbal behavior in a key article published in 1959, and objected to Skinner's somewhat simplistic approach to language learning. In *Syntactic Structures* Chomsky (1957), wrote of linguistic competence, that is, the ideal speaker-listener in the ideal linguistic community. He steered us away from thinking of language acquisition and use as behavior that is learned through instrumental conditioning, toward the notion of language as a cognitive phenomenon.

Speech and language pathologists during the mid-1960's and early 1970's applied aspects of both Chomskian grammar and Skinnerian behaviorism in the assessment and treatment of childhood language disorders. Laura Lee (1966), for example, proposed the protocol of Developmental Sentence Types as a means of measuring the transformational complexity of children's utterances. At the same time that language pathologists and psycholinguists were attempting to refine their approaches to the study and remediation of language, the influence of behaviorism was becoming widespread in the clinical domain. In part urged by the calling to be "accountable" for clinical endeavors, clinicians used the principles of behavior modification to structure their therapy sessions and to quantify observable behaviors. During the mid-1960's and early 1970's, therefore, there appeared a number of high structured and standardized language tests, some of which have been used to study the relation between language and fluency in children. Many of these tests focused primarily on the syntactic aspects of language, such as the Northwestern Syntax Screening Test (Lee, 1971). Other tests tapped syntactic-semantic aspects of language, such as the Test of Auditory Comprehension of Language (Carrow, 1973) and the Carrow Elicited Language Inventory (Carrow, 1974).

Concurrent with the behaviorist orientation in language therapy, psychologists and linguists continued their pursuit of the cognitive bases for language acquisition. There was a resurgence of interest in the works by Jean Piaget, and some pivotal papers (e.g., Bransford and McCarrell, 1972) began to argue for the validity of a cognitive approach to studying language. Even though Chomsky's transformational grammar is no longer considered to be a viable approach to the understanding of language use, we owe a great deal to him and his contemporaries (e.g., Slobin, McNeill, Lenneberg) for inducing us to view language acquisition as, at least in part, a cognitive phenomenon.

Post-Chomsky Trends in the Study of Child Language

A number of very important developments have taken place since the early 1970's, both as a response to Chomskian grammar and as a reaction against it. The cumulative effects of these trends have taken the field of child language to its current forefront. The trends that have evolved in the past decade, summarized here, have dramatically changed the study and treatment of developmental psycholinguistics. It may not be sheer coincidence that the development of fluency also reaches a critical juncture during the very period that language development is at its most active period, namely, the preschool years of childhood.

Greater Emphasis on the Role of Cognitive Development in Language Acquisition   Psycholinguists are fond of saying that language "maps onto" or encodes a child's existing knowledge about the world. Knowledge during these early years consists not of a catalogue of facts, such as the important dates in history, but of the salient concepts and relationships in the environment that are induced by the learner. These relationships revolve around persons, objects, and actions, and emanate from certain Piagetian mental schemas that function as the precursors to language development (Bloom and Lahey, 1978). An example of a mental schema is object permanence, the realization that objects exist separate from and independent of the child's sensorimotor activities as well as of the time and space contexts of the object. Only if a young child understands that objects can exist even if not experiencing their physical presence can he or she begin to generalize names of objects and categorize objects belonging to the same class. The resurgence of interest in Piagetian psychology has had a profound impact on shaping this trend.

Greater Emphasis on the Development of Semantics and Pragmatics in the Study of Child Language   The realization that children's early utterances, if not also later utterances, are motivated by semantic intentions (Bloom, 1970; Schlesinger, 1974) and pragmatic functions (Prutting, 1979) rather than simply syntactic considerations, represented a major turning point. Language pathologists began to realize the imprudence of studying child language from the adult perspective, which had heavily favored syntactic considerations. Although syntax is of course important as a vehicle for language, and although it is difficult to separate syntax from semantics and pragmatics in natural discourse (and indeed we should strive for the well-tuned integration of all three areas), language development during the formative years may be motivated more by semantic and pragmatic than by syntactic concerns.

Pragmatic concerns should be of particular interest for clinicians treating childhood stuttering because the degree of communicative stress has been shown to influence the amount and severity of stuttering (Bloodstein, 1981). We have also observed that the degree of propositionality in a message influences amount of stuttering (e.g., Eisenson and Horowitz, 1945). Eisenson (1975) defined a proposition as "a unit of intellectually meaningful linguistic content" (p. 417) and postulated that "many if not most stutterers experience difficulty in communication, in saying something meaningful and expected in terms of the overall situation. From our point of view, stuttering will not be understood unless we evaluate the linguistic component in the speaking situation" (pp. 417–418). In these terms, then, the current emphases on semantics or the meaning or meaningfulness of utterances, and pragmatics or the functions of utterances in the speaking situation, play key roles in the study of the relation between language and fluency.

Greater Emphasis on a Low Structured Approach to Language Assessment and Therapy   The current use of low structured language sampling techniques and therapy is due largely to the realization by Bloom (1967), later more fully expounded by Bloom and Lahey (1978), that contextual variables are highly critical, both for the child and from the clinician's viewpoint. The meaning of an utterance varies as a function of the pragmatic context of the message. Many high structured tests are devoid of meaningful context for either the stimuli or the child's response, and some scholars postulate that high structured standardized tests can underestimate a child's actual linguistic ability (e.g., Prutting, Gallagher, and Mulac, 1975). The ultimate goal of language assessment is to ascertain the child's representative language abilities, neither under- nor overestimating his linguistic functioning. A low structured naturalistic approach to language assessment and therapy would be vacuous, however, if the linguistic behaviors being assessed or the therapy strategies and goals were not "structured" and well formulated in the clinician's mind. As additional information is gathered on normal language development, such as the form and content categories developed by Bloom and Lahey (1978), we can be increasingly confident in the direction we should take in dealing with children whose language is suspect.

Use of Normal Language Development as a Model for Assessing and Treating Disordered Language Development   Implicit if not explicit in this trend is the realization that the patterns of language development observed in normal youngsters, rather than those observed in adults, should serve as guidelines for diagnostic and therapy strategies. For several decades the norms for gauging whether a child's language is normal were primarily in terms of adult standards (e.g., McCarthy, 1930). By the late 1960's and early 1970's (e.g., Lee, 1966; Miller and Yoder, 1972), however, language pathologists had begun to use normal developmental stages as the bases for assessing and treating language-disordered children. This trend of using normal developmental data to determine language goals is well tuned to the trend toward incorporating a child's cognitive capacities into the treatment designed for his or her language system. That is, speech-language pathologists should be sensitive to the cognitive schemas that are particularly salient for children of different ages.

METHODS OF ASSESSING
DEVELOPMENTAL PSYCHOLINGUISTICS

The popularity of low structured language sampling techniques was noted earlier. However, analysis of language samples is by no means the only approach to the assessment of child language. Approaches to language assessment, whether for clinical or for research purposes, can be schematized along several dimensions—high structured versus low structured, receptive versus expressive, and focus of the test (i.e., on syntax, semantics, pragmatics, or phonology).

High structured tests impose a degree of structure on the testing situation, in terms of both the stimuli from the clinician and the response sought from the child. Typical of high structured tests are standardized, published tests such as the revised PPVT (Dunn, 1981). Not all high structured tests need be published. Clinicians and researchers often construct their own protocols, using techniques such as sentence elicitation tasks, to assess a child's language skills.

Low structured testing attempts to capture the child's language in a naturalistic environment without a structured, preconceived set of stimuli, and is exemplified by the corpus. The major advantage of naturalistic language sampling is the availability of meaningful contexts to give substance and pragmatic motivations to the child's messages. Especially for the very young child, the use of rich interpretation is highly illuminating if not essential to determine the particular syntactic, semantic, or pragmatic nature of the child's utterances. The model often used to determine the adequacy of the child's language follows normal language development, such as Roger Brown's stages (Brown, 1973) or Bloom and Lahey's phases (Bloom and Lahey, 1978).

Receptive language tests tap children's comprehension skills, and expressive language tests attempt to analyze a child's ability to encode language. Often implicit in expressive tasks, however, is also the child's ability to process and understand language, because a child's utterance is seldom elicited without verbal input from the clinician. Tests vary in their emphasis on the particular aspects of language being assessed. Language sampling techniques attempt to assess the interaction of all areas of language—syntax, semantics, pragmatics, and at times phonology. The higher the structure of the test, the more difficult it is to capture all aspects of language, particularly pragmatics. Psycholinguists realize full well that children's early utterances are motivated by their perceptual and cognitive domains, which translate more directly into the semantics and pragmatics of utterances.

Regardless of the type of assessment procedure used, three issues are critical to the usefulness of the results obtained from a test, and all three are important in the study of the relation between language and fluency in children. First is the degree of reliability and validity of the test, that is, the consistency and the "truthfulness," respectively, of the test. The validity of a language test rests heavily on its theoretical orientation, our second issue. The Illinois Tests of Psycholinguistic Abilities (ITPA) (Kirk, McCarthy, and Kirk, 1968), for example, is based on Osgood's model of communication and measures various psycholinguistic processes (receptive and expressive) using different modalities at the representational or automatic level. As theoretical orientations shift in a field, so do the approaches to assessment. The ITPA, for example, is now not considered to be a highly valid language test, although it may tap other important parameters of perceptual and cognitive behaviors (Siegel, 1979). The onus is on the individual professional to keep abreast of the field, to sift through the current literature in the context of the past, and to arrive at a prudent concept of language and, accordingly, a language assessment tool of best fit.

The final issue relates to whether the language test is used in a cross-sectional or a longitudinal study. Cross-sectional studies measure the language skills of a large group of children of different ages at one time; longitudinal studies measure the language skills of a smaller group of children in great detail as the children progress in age. Longitudinal studies are time-consuming, but the type of data obtained is quite rich and valuable. In fact, we need more data based on longitudinal studies.

THE RELATION BETWEEN FLUENCY AND LANGUAGE DEVELOPMENT IN CHILDHOOD

The conjoining of the two fields of developmental psycholinguistics and childhood fluency disorders is attributable to at least two forces. First is the recent surge of interest in and refinement of the study of developmental psycholinguistics, as discussed earlier. The second comes from the growing realization that the various aspects of communication, heretofore dealt within a more or less piecemeal fashion, should be considered as parts of an integrated, synergistic system.

When the subcomponents of the system are in tune, the child's communication system is on its way to normal development. This section reviews what we know about the system, using as the focal point the interplay between children's language development and their fluency. Is there a relation between language development and fluency? If so, what is it? Are there certain variables, such as the age of the child or the severity of the disfluencies, that are particularly influential in molding this relationship? Does the relation between language development and fluency differ for children with so-called normal nonfluencies and those who stutter? How does the relation between fluency and language manifest itself as a function of specific aspects of language, such as syntax, semantics, and pragmatics?

Some Early Studies

At least a surface interest in the relation between speech-language development and fluency existed as early as the 1940's, when researchers found some degree of correlation or observed some linkage between speech-language development and stuttering. Regardless of the strength of the linkage observed, the field of psycholinguistics did not emerge for another 15 or so years, and data from these very early studies should be viewed in that light. Both the theoretical framework and the methodologies for studying language behaviors were at a bare minimum.

The investigators who had some interest in the relation between language and fluency thought of language development primarily as the emergence of first words and sentences or as a syntactic phenomenon, focusing mostly on the length and somewhat on the complexity of utterances (Davis, 1939, 1940). Words were studied in terms of their grammatical class or part of speech, or in terms of the scope of the child's vocabulary as measured by the PPVT.

Representative of this early approach to the investigation of the relation of language to fluency are the studies by Berry (1938), Davis (1939, 1940), Johnson (in Johnson and Leutenegger, 1955), and Metraux (1950). Davis (1939) and Metraux (1950) observed a reduction in syllable, word, and phrase repetitions as children reached 4 and 5 years of age when, presumably, their language sophistication becomes more mature. Davis (1940) further reported a slightly negative correlation between speech repetitions and mean length of response, as well as a rank ordering of speaking situations that produced the most repetitions. At the top of this ranking were speaking when excited over an activity, when wanting to direct the activities of another child, when attempting to attract the attention of another child, when forced by the teacher to change one's own activity, and when upholding one's status in spite of another child. We come back to these speech acts as they relate to a child's fluency later in the chapter. Berry found that young stutterers showed slower speech development compared to nonstutterers. In contrast, the Iowa Studies (Johnson and Leutenegger, 1955) showed that emergence of first words and sentences was comparable for stutterers and nonstutterers based on parental recollection.

Although Brown's studies (1937, 1938, 1945) focused on adult stutterers during the task of oral reading, the work deserves attention here because of 1) its tremendous influence in spurring interest in the relation between language and fluency in adults, and 2) the possible implications such studies on older (adult) stutterers may hold when compared with similar loci studies on younger children. For example, the findings by Brown on adults seem to be corroborated in loci studies of older children who are disfluent (e.g., Williams, Silverman, and Kools, 1969), but not in studies of preschoolers either at the incipient stages of stuttering or when undergoing normal fluency development.

In his seminal work on the loci of stuttering during oral reading by adults, Brown (1945) found that the focal points for stuttering are determined by four so-called word-bound factors: the grammatical class of the word, its position in the utterance, the sound the word begins with, and the length of the word. In particular, stuttering seems to occur more on content words (nouns, verbs, adjectives, adverbs) than on function words such as articles, prepositions, and conjunctions. Moreover, stuttering predominates on words that begin with consonants (other than t, h, w, voiced th) than on vowels, more on words toward or at the beginning of utterances, more on words that are five letters long or longer, and more on the initial sound of a syllable. These findings have been subjected to various interpretations, including explanations based on the grammatical factor, word-bound effects, degree of propositionality or conspicuousness of words, the prosodic attributes of words, and the degree of information load presumed to be contained in the word.

The grammatical class factor refers to the finding that certain grammatical parts of speech, notably those falling in the content category such as nouns and verbs, seem to trigger more stuttering in adults compared to the ."little" words of the function category such as articles and prepositions. Other word-bound effects yielded by Brown's studies indicated that stutterers tend to be disfluent at or toward the beginning of words or utterances. This tendency for the loci of blocks to occur toward the beginning of utterances has been found for phrases (Taylor, 1966) as well as "phonemic clauses," defined by Soderberg (1967) as utterances marked by a primary stress and ending with a terminal juncture.

Brown himself interpreted his findings within the framework of Johnson's evaluation theory of stuttering. That is, fluency failure occurs when the speaker evaluates or perceives difficulty with a particular utterance. The parts of an utterance that are the most salient, contribute the most meaning, or occur at the beginning of an utterance are the most conspicuous. The saliency of these features, in turn, instills anxiety in the speaker.

> *It is probably in terms of the evaluation of words as being conspicuous, prominent, or meaningful that the loci of stutterings are to be accounted for, rather than directly in terms of the sheer presence or absence of any factor or factors. The significance of such evaluation of a word by the stutterer appears to lie in the fact that having so evaluated a word, he desires to avoid stuttering on it. He reacts accordingly with caution, hesitancy, effort, conflict, etc.—and it is predominantly these reactions which are termed stuttering, as contrasted with "normal" or nonstuttering speech interruptions* (Brown, 1945, p. 192).

As reflected in the quotation above, Brown focused his interpretations on the word-bound effects of stuttering, the attributes triggering stuttering that are specific to the lexical item rather than to the entire utterance or to the syllable.

In his study relating stuttering to "word accent," Brown (1938) found that stuttering tends to occur on stressed syllables of words. He interpreted this finding also in terms of the relative conspicuousness of linguistic stress. Wingate (1977, 1979) believed that this latter finding by Brown deserved greater attention in the literature, stating that ". . . the relationship between linguistic stress and stuttering continues to be the most important bit of information that has yet been found in the research on linguistic factors in stuttering" (1977, p. 47). Wingate pointed to the coincidental overlapping of the various word-bound factors with the prosodic features of linguistic stress. For example, stress during connected speech often falls on the more important content words than on function words such as articles and prepositions. Moreover, the central role of linguistic stress in stuttering should be couched in physiological terms and, more specifically, in phonatory rather than psychological terms.

To put the matter simply, execution of stress prominences in the speech stream is essentially a phonatory function; that is, the expression of linguistic stress is a function of an increased energizing of several actions fundamental to phonation. It should be noted that this explanation clearly reflects a performance (i.e., motor, physiological) difficulty rather than a reactive (i.e., psychological) one (Wingate, 1977, p. 48).

In addition to examining the loci data from a prosodic perspective as Wingate has done, other researchers have interpreted the data in terms of the information value of words. Words containing high information load carry the least amount of redundancy and predictability based on the technique of forward guessing of words in an utterance. Using this technique, we have found that content words and words at the beginning of utterances are often associated with high information value. An everyday illustration is the typical telegram, which contains primarily content words rather than the relatively less significant function words.

It must be emphasized that the studies by Brown were based on adults during oral reading tasks, not on children nor during spontaneous, natural discourse. Nonetheless, this work is discussed because of its role in directing researchers' attention to the possible relations between linguistic features of utterances and fluency. Moreover, a review of this work allows us to juxtapose the set of data on older children and adults with the research that continues to be conducted on young children. Some interesting patterns are beginning to emerge as a function of whether the stutterer is a preschooler, a child of elementary school age, or an adult. We now review findings from some current studies on the relation between language and fluency behavior in children.

Some More Current Studies

These studies are organized in terms of the methodologies used to capture the language and language-related skills as they pertain to children's development of fluency. The methodologies include studies based on case history information or surveys, language sampling techniques, and standardized testing or other high structured testing protocols.

In each subsection based on the three methodological approaches, studies are discussed wherever possible according to the age of the children. The chapter concludes with discussion of the state of the art of our knowledge about the relation between language and fluency.

Studies Based on Case History Information or Surveys   Two of the most often quoted studies designed to tap the onset and nature of childhood stuttering in general, and yielding some insight about the relation of stuttering and speech-language development in particular, have been the cross-sectional studies done in the midwestern United States by Johnson and Associates (1959) and the cross-sectional and longitudinal studies of children from Newcastle-upon-Tyne, England, by Andrews and Harris (1964) and Morley (1967). In addition to the intrinsic difference in methodology between cross-sectional and longitudinal studies, these surveys also differ depending on whether the data were collected based on in situ observations by the experimenter or on a review of case histories of children. In some instances, survey studies are conducted by interviewing parents on their recollections of past and observations of present behaviors in their children.

The Iowa Studies, based largely on interviews with parents and case history information, were conducted by Wendell Johnson and his associates. Although parents of the stutterers perceived their children's speech development as "much slower than average," the data showed no statistically significant differences in speech development between the two groups. For example, the mean ages for speaking first words and first sentences, respectively, were 10.8 and 21 months for the control group, and 10.9 and 21.8 months for the experimental group. The types of information sought by Johnson and his colleagues regarding the children's speech and language development included questions on the amount of talking the children did, vocabulary and grammar skills, and amount of talking allowed at the dinner table. The two groups of children, based on findings of Study III of the Iowa Studies, were "essentially alike" in the various aspects of speech development and speech-language behaviors. In contrast, the data gathered by Andrews and Harris (1964) and Morley (1967) at Newcastle-upon Tyne showed greater delay in speech and language development for the stutterers. In comparing differences between stuttering and nonstuttering groups of children, Andrews and Harris wrote:

An expected finding which is consistent with other work in the field was that stutterers were some four months retarded in the acquisition of first phrases, and that, when they did talk, considerably more of them suffered from articulatory defects, usually of a developmental nature. Stutterers, then, tend to be "late and poor" talkers, both findings being significant at the 1 per cent level (Andrews and Harris, 1964, p. 72).

More recently, Williams and Silverman (1968) compared 115 stutterers and nonstutterers based on speech-language examination and found the incidence of other speech defects (particularly misarticulations) to be higher for the stutterers (23.5%) than for the nonstutterers (8.7%). Based on questionnaires filled out by clinicians on more than 1,000 school-aged stutterers from 31 states, Blood and Seider (1981) determined that 10% of the stutterers had some kind of language problem and 11% had articulatory defects.

Studies Based on Language Sampling Techniques The use of language sampling is at once a very traditional as well as a very current assessment approach. Except for a hiatus during the 1960's when standardized language testing was very much in vogue, partly because of the popularity of behaviorism, language sampling has withstood the test of time, undoubtedly reflecting the richness of data that can be obtained from detailed analyses of the corpus. The potential for richness of data retrieval and analysis becomes increasingly well realized as the field of psycholinguistics itself advanced. Davis (1939, 1940) conducted some of the earliest works using the method of analyzing children's language in natural environments. In addition to the previously mentioned finding of a slightly negative correlation between speech repetitions and mean length of response, Davis also found some situational variables that affected the amount of nonfluencies in her normal preschoolers. The highest rate of repetition behavior was provoked when the child was excited and when the child wanted to control another child's behavior; the situation that least provoked repetition behavior was offering information to the teacher. These data were gathered from 62 preschoolers in two half-hour sessions of free play "when teacher-domination was at a minimum."

Comparing the language samples of kindergarteners and first graders, E.-M. Silverman and Williams (1967) found that stutterers were slightly poorer in mean length of response, mean of the five longest responses, and the structural complexity of utterances. Colburn and Mysak (1982) analyzed the speech samples of four preschoolers in a longitudinal study as the children progressed from successive single-word utterances to the emergence of syntax. A major purpose of the study was to trace the covariation of normal fluency development and normal language acquisition as measured by mean length of utterance (MLU) and the occurrence of specific semantic-syntactic structures. Although widespread differences existed between subjects, any given child's profile of fluency disruptions showed systematic changes as a function of the maturation of specific semantic-syntactic structures. The nonfluencies appeared to be particulary closely associated with the semantic-syntactic structures that were undergoing development. Colburn and Mysak attributed these temporary disruptions of fluency to a "practicing effect," a potentially interesting construct that deserves further empirical research. One of the findings from the study was that "developmental disfluency appeared to attach itself to structures that were learned and used regularly, reflecting practicing of that structure" (p. 424) rather than on novel structures, as had been anticipated.

The bulk of the work using language sampling as the preferred method of research has studied the distribution of disfluencies in children's spontaneous utterances. These studies, spurred directly or indirectly from the early data on adults by Brown, compared the frequency and loci of occurrence of disfluencies in children. Recall that Brown's data on adults during oral reading showed the loci of stuttering to be associated with content words, words at or toward the initial position of utterances, words beginning with consonants, and longer words. The research using language sampling on children thus far seems to show a developmental pattern whereby, regardless of whether the children are diagnosed as stutterers, there seems to be a greater demarcation between the preschool child and the child of elementary school age than between the older child and the adult.

Bloodstein and Gantwerk (1967) analyzed the spontaneous speech of 13 young stutterers ages 2 to 6 years and found that the disfluencies occurred on all parts of speech but, in particular, on pronouns and conjunctions. These results may at first be interpreted in a grammatical factor framework (i.e., specific parts of speech are especially prone to stuttering). Bloodstein and Gantwerk were quick to point out, however, that the high occurrence of stuttering on conjunctions and pronouns is really attributable to a positional effect, because these two parts of speech occur frequently at the beginning of utterances.

In an article on the rules of early stuttering, Bloodstein (1974) reexamined the language samples of six stutterers, ages 3 to 6 years, and reaffirmed the notion that loci of early stuttering occur at the beginning of utterances. He interpreted these findings according to the theory that stuttering emanates from tension and results in the fragmentation of "higher-order constituents" (i.e., syntactic units) rather than specific words. These results were again confirmed in the study by Bloodstein and Grossman (1981) on the free speech of five preschool stutterers, who tended to stutter at the beginning of sentences and clauses. Moreover, most of the subjects stuttered proportionately more on function than on content words, and more on monosyllabic than on polysyllabic words.

Congruent with the above-mentioned studies were results reported by Wall, Starkweather, and Cairns (1981), which found significantly more stuttering for nine stutterers ages 4 to 6 years at clause boundaries than at internal or nonboundary positions of clauses. Moreover, the conjunction "and" at the beginning of simple and complex sentences was associated with a high rate of stuttering.

Whereas the foregoing studies focused on the loci of stuttering in preschool stutterers, a handful of studies have also looked at the distribution of nonfluencies in normal preschoolers. Helmreich and Bloodstein (1973) examined the language samples of 15 normal preschoolers (mean age of 4 years 4 months) and found no particular tendency for the subjects to be disfluent on nouns, verbs, adjectives, and adverbs. However, pronouns and conjunctions incurred significantly large amounts of fluency disruptions. Based on the similarities in findings between the normal youngsters in this study and the preschool stutterers examined by Bloodstein and Gantwerk (1967), the authors' viewpoint was that the results upheld the validity of the continuity hypothesis.

Based largely on detailed analyses of the speech samples of 10 nonstuttering 4-year-old boys in two types of speaking situation, E.-M. Silverman reported some results that are of interest for comparison between younger and older children. The types of fluency behavior considered were interjections of sound and syllable, part-word repetitions, whole-word repetitions, disrhythmic phonation, and tense pauses. The first of two speaking situations was a preschool classroom in which subjects were interacting with familiar people, participating in structured small and large group activities. In the second speaking situation, a structured interview, subjects were interacting with an experimenter by telling stories based on picture cards, answering questions from the experimenter, and answering questions about themselves and their families. The following results were reported:

1. Although the distribution of the duration and extent of nonfluency types was similar for the two speaking situations, there were more nonfluencies in the structured interview (Silverman, 1972a).

2. There was a preponderance of word repetitions in the subjects' speech samples and little relation between fluency and measures of language behavior (Silverman, 1972b) .

3. Subjects produced nearly twice as many disfluencies in single instances compared to runs/clusters (i.e., disfluencies on the same word and/or consecutive words) for both speaking situations, although subjects produced more disfluencies in runs than would be expected by chance (Silverman, 1973a).

4. There were more nonfluencies on pronouns and conjunctions relative

to other parts of speech and more nonfluencies on the first words of utterances (Silverman, 1974).

5. There was no evidence of a phonetic factor (i.e., more nonfluencies on consonants compared to vowels) in either speaking situations (Silverman, 1975).

In another paper also based on the speech samples of these 10 normal 4-year-olds taken in the classroom setting, Silverman (1973b) found that 1) subjects were more nonfluent during socialized than during egocentric speech, 2) the nonfluency levels during egocentric speech varied as a function of the particular type of egocentric speech produced such that subjects were more nonfluent during dual monologue (considered by Piaget to be the most socialized of the various types of egocentric speech) than during either monologue or echolalic speech, and 3) subjects were more nonfluent for the types of socialized utterance considered to be conveying "adapted information" (i.e., informing or influencing the listener) than for those considered to be "emotionally toned" (e.g., "Gee!" "There!"). Based on the latter finding, it was concluded that there may be a parallel between normally nonfluent children, such as Silverman's subjects, and incipient stutterers. That is, both groups show more fluency disruptions under communicative pressure or stress, as when having to adapt to or influence the listener.

Analyzing the spontaneous speech of 110 Norwegian preschoolers (2 stutterers and 108 nonstutterers), Bjerkan (1980) also found that fluency behaviors reflected the social situational context of the utterances. In particular, many of the repetitions of the younger subjects in the study consisted of reiterating demands that had not been responded to the first time or attempting to attract the attention of the listener. Bjerkan found that repetitions decreased with increasing age, particularly around the period when subjects' MLU reached 3.5 to 4.5.

Muma (1971) was one of the first to systematically analyze the syntactic aspects of preschoolers' fluency behavior using the framework of transformational grammar. The language samples of 26 nonstuttering 4-year-olds (13 called "highly fluent" and 13 "highly disfluent") were transcribed. These samples were taken during the children's description and discussion of the Children's Apperception Test (CAT) pictures by Bellak and Bellak (1959). Muma found that the fluent group used significantly more double-base transformations (complex sentences) than did the less fluent group. Applying a constituent structure analysis to the language samples of four 5- and 6-year-old male stutterers and four controls, Wall (1980) found that the stutterers generally used fewer clauses than the nonstutterers for the same number of words, and used fewer complex sentences, complement clauses, and coordinate clauses. Finally, in a graduate thesis at Brooklyn College cited by Bloodstein (1981), Sichel (1973) found that normal preschoolers were somewhat more disfluent on initial vowels than on initial consonants. However, these results may have been attributable in part to the frequent repetitions of "and" at the beginning of sentences and clauses.

In a study of older normal and stuttering youngsters, Berryman and Kools (1975) found no relation between nonfluency and judges' ratings of language level, reading ability, or intelligence for the 92 first graders examined. In an earlier investigation, Perozzi and Kunze (1969) had used both formal testing (ITPA) and various measures based on subjects' language samples (e.g., mean length of response and structural complexity index) on 10 second grade and 10 third grade stutterers and their controls. The only statistically significant difference between the normals and the stutterers was the Visual-Motor Sequencing subtest of the ITPA, in favor of the controls. In their study of 76 stutterers and 76 controls ranging from kindergarteners through the sixth graders, Williams, Silverman, and Kools (1969) found influences for the loci of stuttering for these older elementary school children similar to those reported earlier for adults.

Studies Based on High Structured Tests or Testing Protocols   Researchers have also resorted to the use of high structured and/or standardized tests or testing protocols to study the relation between fluency and language. As before, the studies are reviewed roughly according to the age of children studied.

Using the PPVT, the Northwestern Syntax Screening Test, and the verbal section of the Preschool Language Scale, Murray and Reed (1977) found that their preschool stutterers scored lower than their respective controls. Kline and Starkweather (1979) used both standardized tests and an analysis of children's MLU, and found that the preschool stutterers performed more poorly than the nonstutterers in their expressive as well as receptive language skills. Moreover, there was high correlation between the receptive and expressive measures. An interpretation from these results is that the children's depressed expressive language measures perhaps reflected linguistic competence, not merely their use of shorter sentences to avoid stuttering.

On the other hand, Haynes and Hood (1977) did not find a meaningful relation between Developmental Sentence Scoring (DSS) scores and either the eight disfluency types analyzed or total number of disfluencies in the 4-, 6-, and 8-year-old nonstutterers they studied. However, the youngsters' overall disfluencies decreased and the predominant types of disfluency changed as the subjects' linguistic skills increased.

In a study of kindergarteners and first graders, Westby (1979) found that stutterers and nonstutterers performed comparably when their respective language samples were analyzed according to the DSS. However, the stutterers performed worse than controls on the standardized tests of the PPVT and the Torrance Test of Creative Thinking, a task tapping semantic divergent thinking. Two studies using the ITPA found some differentiation in performance between young stutterers and nonstutterers. Stocker and Parker (1977) found 4- to 11-year-old stutterers performing worse than nonstutterers on the Sequential Memory subtest of the ITPA and on the Auditory Attention Subtest for Related Syllables of the Detroit Tests of Learning Aptitude. Based on a study of 28 stutterers (5 to 9 years old), Williams and Marks (1972) reported some depression in the auditory-vocal sequencing skills relative to the overall ITPA profile of the subjects. Moreover, there was a tendency toward weakness at the automatic level, particularly with the auditory-vocal sequencing skills.

Structured language assessment has not been limited to standardized testing, and several researchers have devised their own ways of manipulating the language variables to observe their impact on children's fluency. Pearl and Bernthal (1980) studied the effect of grammatical complexity on the nonfluency of 30 nonstutterers 3 to 4 years of age, with MLU ranging from 2.06 to 6.30. These children were judged by the experimenters to have normal articulation and language, and they had scored above the 25th percentile on the Northwestern Syntax Screening Test. Tape recordings of 30 sentences representing 6 different grammatical constructions, but all containing 6 to 8 morphemes (or syllables), were presented to the subjects to repeat. Results indicated individual differences across subjects' nonfluencies as influenced by sentence types. More than half the nonfluencies made by the five most fluent children occurred on sentences that were correctly imitated, in contrast to the five most nonfluent children, who made 80% of their nonfluencies on sentences that were incorrectly imitated. Pearl and Bernthal interpreted this as support for the "grammatical complexity/disfluency hypothesis" (i.e., there is a relation between disfluency and imitation errors of sentences of varying grammatical complexity), at least for the subjects who were relatively more nonfluent. However, according to the investigators, factors other than grammatical complexity probably influenced the nonfluency behavior of the relatively more fluent preschool children.

Using a similar technique of sentence elicitations but on 40 normal kindergarteners, Haynes and Hood (1978) modeled simple sentences (extensions of basic kernel sentences without major transformations) and complex sentences as the children viewed pictures. The complex sentences were considered to be within the subjects' linguistic capability, and length of sentences was controlled as complexity increased. Results indicated that: 1) the total instances of nonfluencies per 100 words were significantly higher in the complex modeling condition; 2) there were more nonfluencies in the complex modeling situation that were word repetitions, revision-incomplete phrases, and disrhythmic phonation; and 3) the children differed in their points of fluency breakdown. Using 10 nonstutterers, aged

5 years, Gordon (1982) found significant differences in the number of disfluencies occurring in various types of sentence construction for the sentence-modeling task, but not for the sentence-imitation task. The sentence-modeling task consisted of showing each child a picture frame containing two pictorial examples of a syntactic construction. The child was required to model the syntactic construction for the second picture following the examiner's example for the first picture.

Bernstein (1981) analyzed the elicited language of eight stutterers and eight normally fluent preschool through second grade children with the mean age of 6 years for both groups. In the context of a Language Lotto game, the children were asked to assign captions to cartoon pictures. Only full sentences (those containing noun phrase–auxiliary–verb phrase) were considered. There was a significant difference in degree of disfluency between the two groups, with hesitations constituting the most frequent form of disfluency for both groups, and disfluencies occurring significantly more often at constituent-internal loci for stutterers than for the nonstutterers.

The paradigm of verbal reaction time has been used by experimental psychologists to probe subjects' skills in vocabulary storage and retrieval. In an object-naming task in which 8 male stutterers and 20 male nonstutterers (mean age of 8 years for both groups) were asked to name 34 pictures of objects whose names ranged from high to low frequency of occurrence, Boysen and Cullinan (1971) found no difference in reaction time between the two groups of children.

The last two studies to be considered under the category of structured (but nonstandardized) assessment techniques used to study the relation between language and fluency attempted to examine the ability to process and manipulate speech sounds in older children. Perozzi (1970) gave the Tiffany Backward Speech Test (task consists of reversing sounds in a spoken word) to 20 stutterers and 20 nonstutterers of elementary school age. Although the mean score was lower for the stutterers than for the nonstutterers, the difference was not statistically significant. Results were interpreted in terms of the "sound-mindedness" hypothesis (Tiffany, 1963; Wingate, 1967). Manning and Riensche (1976) did not find significant overall difference between 30 stutterers and 30 nonstutterers from 5 to 10 years of age on a task to tap the children's "auditory assembly ability." Subjects were asked to repeat both meaningful and nonmeaningful CVC syllables with varying silent interphonemic intervals of 100, 200, 300, and 400 msec. The two groups of children did not differ in performance. Thus these results do not seem to implicate selected skills required for the auditory processing or auditory-vocal processing of verbal input. However, we know very little about the nature and implications of auditory-vocal processing, and interpretations of research results must be held in abeyance.

Skills tapped by the ITPA (Stocker and Parker, 1977), for example, may not be equatable with skills tapped by tasks in the Tiffany Backward Speech Test.

A final group of investigators have attempted to search for a relation between reading skills and fluency patterns in subjects of mid- and late childhood years. Silverman and Williams (1973) asked 135 second through sixth graders (69 stutterers and 66 nonstutterers) to read from readers one year below grade level. Interestingly they found that the nonstutterers revised a higher percentage (40%) of their reading errors than did the stutterers, even though the groups made comparable numbers of reading errors. Based on results from 80 normal third through sixth graders reading passages of different difficulty levels, Cecconi, Hood, and Tucker (1977) found a significant increase in disfluency as reading difficulty level increased. Moreover, there was a tendency for an increase in the disfluency types typically associated with stuttering (e.g., part-word repetitions, disrhythmic phonation, tense pauses) as reading difficulty increased. The authors speculated that a strong link exists between language and reading skills on disfluency, particularly when the demands for a child's linguistic expression exceed his capacity.

FLUENCY AND LANGUAGE: A SYNTHESIS

Thus far we have surveyed the current trends in the field of child language, discussed various methodological approaches to the study of developmental psycholinguistics, and summarized the available information on the relation between language and fluency, organized according to methodological approaches used in the research. Let us stand back for a moment and try to extract any patterns that may surface from the data and examine some variables that are particularly pertinent to our interpretation of this growing corpus of data. The chapter concludes with some thoughts about the relation between language and fluency in childhood, and comments on the implications of this relation for the assessment and treatment of childhood stuttering as well as for future research.

The generalizations on the relation between fluency and language that follow are based on the state of the art. Some of the generalizations stand on research findings that have been replicated by various investigators, such as the observation that disfluencies occur at the beginning of utterances for preschoolers. Other generalizations are much more tenuous and are offered as hypotheses in need of further investigation.

The Relation between Fluency and Language

Some Precautionary Notes

1.   Particularly because there are multiple facets of linguistic behaviors, generalizations regarding the relation between fluency and language must be couched in the context of one's definition of language.

2.   Patterns on the relation between fluency and language become anomalous when examining results of high structured standardized tests. The variability of these results may reflect essential or intrinsic differences in subjects' language skills, but may also reflect the definition and scope of the language being tapped by the particular test. That is, high structured standardized tests differ in their theoretical definitions of language, in the particular aspects of language being measured, and in their degrees of validity and reliability.

3.   The parceling of spheres of influence to the various areas of language (i.e., syntax, semantics, and pragmatics) becomes increasingly difficult and impractical the more "naturalistic" the language sampling technique used.

General Patterns

1.   There seems to be some delay in speech-language development for at least a proportion of children diagnosed as stutterers.

2.   The age of the child seems to be a key variable in determining the strength and nature of this relationship, particularly in studies determining the distribution of fluency breakdowns in the stream of linguistic utterances.

3.   Studies on normal fluency development (reviewed by Starkweather, 1980) have shown that type and amount of fluency behavior change as the child gets older. Such changes may be evidenced at a macroscopic level (e.g., a general decline in certain types of nonfluency with an overall increase in speech rate). At a more microscopic level Colburn and Mysak (1982) found greater fluency for a particular semantic-syntactic structure as that structure is being acquired during the preschool years.

4.   Differences may exist in individual children's fluency behavior as a function of the degrees of linguistic load placed on the child at different times.

Fluency and Syntax

1.   Syntax has been variously referred to or defined as grammar, parts of speech, the so-called grammatical factor in stuttering, the length and complexity of utterances, the manner in which a child encodes specific semantic categories, and the encoding of an entire grammatical unit (as opposed to smaller units such as syllables or words).

2.   The loci studies have yielded some fairly consistent patterns regarding points of fluency breakdown as a function of grammatical parts of speech.

Interpretations for the various patterns observed in subjects of various ages, however, have differed from investigator to investigator. These explanations have included prosodic influences on stuttering (Wingate, 1976, 1979), the perception at the beginning of an utterance of difficulty in encoding the entire utterance (Bloodstein and Gantwerk, 1967), and information value or points of high uncertainty for the loci of disfluencies (Soderberg, 1967).

The patterns seem to be determined in part by the age of subjects studied. Patterns observed for children of preschool age include the following. First, specific grammatical parts of speech per se do not seem to be the primary determinant of loci of disfluencies; rather, the encoding of larger units such as clauses and phrases seems to occupy this role. However, perhaps because pronouns and conjunctions predominate at the beginning of syntactic units, words of these types also show high prevalence of fluency disruptions for both normal and stuttering preschoolers. Moreover, the foregoing results have been interpreted in the framework of tension and fragmentation of "higher-order constituents of language" (Bloodstein, 1981).

Older children, not unlike adults, experience greater disfluencies on words that: 1) begin with consonants; 2) are content words such as nouns, verbs, adjectives, and adverbs; 3) are relatively long; and 4) occur at or toward the beginning of sentences. These patterns have been interpreted in terms of the greater degree of conspicuousness and meaningfulness or stimulus value that specific words carry for the older child.

3.   Relatively nonfluent children who are nevertheless not considered to be stutterers tend to use sentences that are syntactically simpler than those used by fluent children (Muma, 1971).

4.   Likewise, preschool stutterers tend to use simpler syntactic constructions than those chosen by matched controls.

5.   There seems to be some validity in the notion of "grammatical load" when children are subjected to relatively more complex sentences to model compared to simpler sentences. However, the relation between grammatical complexity and nonfluencies is complicated when the degree of grammatical complexity is controlled for (Pearl and Bernthal, 1980).

Fluency and Semantics

1.   Semantics has generally been thought of as the study of meaning. Meaning, in turn, can be considered in various and more specific ways. If "meaning" is the meaningfulness of words, then a great deal of interest has been shown in the literature in the meaningfulness and degree of information value of words as they are related to the loci of stuttering. "Information value" is a term derived from information theory: a lexical item carries greater information value, or load, if subjects cannot predict that word in contextual speech.

2.   Semantics as it relates to fluency can also be thought of in terms of the propositionality of speech. Semantics in this context is very closely related to the pragmatic aspects of language. Eisenson (1958), for example, points to the reduced propositional value of a passage on repeated readings as an explanation of diminished stuttering. Jakobovits (1966) hypothesized that successful readings of the same words during adaptation tasks reduce the meaning or meaningfulness of words.

3.   Semantics can also be thought of as the maturity of vocabulary acquisition, tapped by such measures as the PPVT. Murray and Reed (1977), for example, found that their preschool stutterers scored lower than matched controls on the PPVT. Hegde (1981) spoke of poor "lexical control" as a "first-order" antecedent of childhood disfluencies in a study of the relation between language and fluency in childhood.

4.   Semantic development can be thought of in terms of the acquisition of semantic-syntactic structures following the framework developed by Bloom and Lahey (1978), as exemplified by the work of Colburn and Mysak (1982), who found systematic changes in the individual fluency profiles of preschoolers as their semantic-syntactic structures emerged. These semantic-syntactic structures include the linguistic coding of action, attribution, existence, and state of relationships. The authors found a temporary "practice effect" during which normal children exhibit greater degrees of nonfluencies as they acquire specific semantic-syntactic structures.

5.   A great deal more research is needed not only to explore but also to define aspects of semantic development that are related to childhood fluency behavior. A child's word-retrieval skills, for example, may be one of many fruitful constructs to study to determine the relation between semantic development and fluency.

Fluency and Pragmatics

1.   Pragmatics has been considered from many vantage points, and various systems have been developed (e.g., Dore, 1975; Halliday, 1974) to systematize aspects of pragmatic behavior.

2.   Children tend to exhibit greater degrees of nonfluency or stuttering when the discourse context contains disruptive and stressful elements. Discourse contexts in which the child attempts to make demands on others, or authority figures make demand on him, seem to be particularly associated with a rise in fluency breakdown.

3.   Normal preschoolers seem to show greater amounts of nonfluencies in speaking situations that require one-to-one interaction, such as a "structured interview" (Silverman, 1972a), compared to discourse in a more naturalistic classroom setting. However, the investigator also should consider other pragmatic variables that interact with the discourse setting, such as the nature of the discourse itself.

4.   Pragmatic interpretations can be applied to Piaget's categories of socialized versus egocentric speech. Socialized speech, according to Piaget, aims to influence or inform the listener. Egocentric speech is devoid of a desire to influence the listener. Using these terminologies, preschoolers tend to be more nonfluent during socialized speech; and within the category of egocentric speech, "dual monologue" has been observed to produce the highest degree of nonfluencies. The explanations for these findings have been interpreted in terms of Bloodstein's continuity hypothesis: "[that] the disfluent behavior of nonstutterers is similar to that of stutterers, namely communicative pressure or stress" (Silverman, 1973b, p. 478).

Fluency and Phonology

1.   Broadly speaking, phonology is the study of the sound system in a language. The clinical application of phonological analyses is one of the more recent developments in our profession as we search for patterns or processes in children's sound system. Childhood phonology is undergoing a good deal of flux as researchers and clinicians attempt to consider it under the overall framework of communication disorders (Shriberg and Kwiatkowski, 1982). If we consider phonology in its broadest sense, as above, then a small handful of studies have examined the relation between fluency and children's ability to perceive or produce sounds in their language.

2.   Although the literature on adults reports a phonetic influence on the occurrence of disfluencies, this has not yet been consistently observed in young children.

3.   It is also difficult to generalize about children's ability at tasks requiring the manipulation of speech sounds. This skill was suspect in a study by Perozzi (1970) in which the mean score on the Tiffany Backward Speech Test was lower for children who stuttered than for the controls. This finding was related to the "sound-mindedness" hypothesis as a factor influencing stuttering.

Fluency and Reading

1.   Although particulars about the relation between reading and language have yet to be delineated, reading itself involves aspects of language processing. Vellutino and Shub, who argue that language is the "dominant system" in reading feel that ". . . success in identifying whole words is especially dependent on the child's familiarity with a word's semantic and syntactic properties, whereas success in phonetic decoding depends primarily on familiarity with its phonological properties" (1982, p. 23).

2.   The few studies that have tried to systematically vary reading level difficulty to determine its effect on fluency seem to point to an increasing rate of disfluency as reading difficulty increases (e.g., Cecconi, Hood, and Tucker, 1977).

3.   However, nonstutterers in one study (Silverman and Williams, 1973) were more prone to correct their own reading errors than were stutterers, even though both groups' reading materials were one year below grade level and the groups made comparable numbers of reading errors.

Some Variables in the Relation between Fluency and Language

In our review of the data available on the relation between language and fluency in childhood, we have attempted to sift out any patterns that may exist. Some patterns were found repeatedly across studies, but many are to be regarded as tentative and embryonic, and in need of a great deal more research.

Now we analyze this body of research from another perspective, one that has implications for future research as well as for clinical management. This vantage point consists of teasing out variables that are likely to make a difference either in an experimental design or in the design of a therapy program for a child who stutters.

Age of the Child   Age seems to be an important variable for the study of the relation between fluency and language. Recall, for example, that for both preschool stutterers and nonstutterers the distribution of disfluencies tends to occur primarily at or near the beginning of utterances such as sentences, clauses, or phrases. A shift in primary loci occurs later in childhood, some say during the early elementary school years, whereupon the loci become associated with smaller units such as words or even specific phonemes. This word-bound effect becomes very evident during adulthood (Brown, 1945).

These findings have been interpreted on the basis of the grammatical factors of words, the greater propositionality of stuttered words, and the greater information load of stuttered words. In addition to these influences, the clinician and researcher should be aware of the influence of some other variables that are likely to be operative, especially during early childhood. These variables include the child's ongoing development of the various levels of his language system. In addition to developing a profile of the child's fluency patterns, the clinician should also draw up a profile of the child's language skills. The language-based therapy approach pre-

sented in this book treats the young stutterer only after careful consideration of both these profiles. The child whose syntactic-semantic development
is not up to par, for example, would be approached differently from the
child with poor pragmatic skills. Not all young stutterers, of course, experience a delay in language. But even for the young stutterer with normally
developing language, the clinician should be attuned to the ramifications
of linguistic loading on the child and should tailor the therapy activities
accordingly.

Another variable to consider is the nature of the child's stuttering as a
function of age. The chapter on symptomatology, for example, discussed
the possibility of subgroups of childhood stutterers and the likelihood of
multiple tracks such as those observed by Van Riper (1982) for the development of stuttering. The episodicity of childhood stuttering even within a
particular time frame, let alone across time frames as the child grows
older, must be considered.

Loci of Disfluencies   Webster's *Seventh New Collegiate Dictionary* defines locus (plural is "loci") as "place, locality, the set of all points whose
location is determined by stated conditions." Applied to stuttering, therefore, "loci" refers to points at which fluency disruptions cluster, for whatever reason.

According to Muma:

> *The underlying assumptions of both the loci and non-loci ap-
> proaches appear to be that certain aspects of grammar evoke a
> psychological breakdown (either emotionally or in process complex-
> ity, such as memory load), resulting in disfluency. The loci approach
> posits that there is a one-to-one correspondence between the psycho-
> logical breakdown and the moment of disfluency, whereas the non-
> loci approach rests on the notion that the moment of disfluency need
> not occur at the same point of psychological breakdown. However,
> there is another side to the coin. That is, both approaches are
> consonant with the notion that disfluency causes a unique change in
> linguistic performance other than, of course, disfluency; for exam-
> ple, speakers may use simpler utterances to compensate for their
> disfluent behaviors*
> (Muma, 1971, p. 428).

Why are we interested in whether there are points in an utterance that
are particularly prone to disfluencies? At least on a descriptive level, we
are interested in researching the patterns that exist in the distribution of
stuttering in children's utterances. At a deeper and more speculative level,
we wish to search for explanations for the patterns observed. Why do these

patterns occur? How are they influenced by other variables, such as those discussed with regard to the age of the child? How could these observations and interpretations fit into an overall model of childhood stuttering?

Although the underlying theme of this chapter has been the psycholinguistic aspects of childhood stuttering, an alternative explanation for the loci of stuttering at the beginnings of clauses and phrases, for example, might ultimately be traced to the co-occurrence of syntactic structures with physiological concomitants.

Level of Communicative Responsibility In keeping with the current trend of considering a child's communicative ability to be a suprastructure for his speech or for his linguistic skills (Prutting, 1982), clinicians in the final analysis must attend to the overall communicative demand of utterances on the child's stuttering. The Stocker Probe Technique (Rev. Ed., 1980) is a diagnostic tool and treatment program for young stutterers that explicitly take into account the communicative responsibility of utterances. According to Stocker, the degree of communicative responsibility or "level of demand" depends on such variables as creativity, and the degree of novelty of and uncertainty about the message. Decreasing the level of demand should decrease the level of creativity, hence increasing the likelihood that the child will become more fluent. In his prefatory notes to the Stocker Probe Technique manual, Jon Eisenson reaffirms his long-held views relating stuttering (and acquired aphasia) to the degree of propositionality of utterances. The role of perceived communicative responsibility may be quite salient in the assessment and treatment of the young disfluent child.

Fluency and the Language-disordered Child Although most of the research reviewed dealt with the relation between language and fluency either in normal children or in youngsters who stutter, a few authors have investigated this relationship in the language-delayed child. Even before the emergence of this issue in the literature, clinicians and clinical supervisors occasionally observed the (temporary) disruption of a child's fluency during treatment for articulation or language disorders. Hall (1977) reported case studies of two language-disordered school-age children who became excessively disfluent as they were receiving speech and language therapy, even though neither client had exhibited abnormal fluency patterns initially. However, the disfluencies decreased substantially as the children's language skills improved.

To investigate the relation between fluency and language in language-disordered children, Merits-Patterson and Reed (1981) studied three groups of nonstuttering youngsters 4 to 6 years of age consisting of: nine language-delayed children receiving language therapy to increase MLU and improve syntactic abilities, nine with normal language development, and nine with language delay but not receiving therapy. Results based on transcripts of children during free speech showed the following: 1) no child in any of the three groups was considered "perfectly fluent," 2) the language-delayed children receiving therapy had significantly more part-word and whole-word repetitions than the other two groups, and 3) the language-delayed nontherapy group did not differ significantly from the control group in disfluency types. The authors concluded, "Language delay, per se, did not affect fluency for the nontherapy experimental group" (Merits-Patterson and Reed, 1981, p. 58). Furthermore, the observation that disfluencies increased for the language therapy group may be due either to the increased language uncertainty that children experience as a function of language therapy or to pragmatic considerations of the therapy milieu that heighten the "communication pressure" or stress.

Fluency and Language Development: Implications for Research and Clinical Management

The research findings reviewed in this chapter point to some important implications for future research and for the clinical management of childhood stuttering. Except for the statement of the need for additional longitudinal studies, these implications apply equally to the laboratory and to the clinic, suggesting the following guidelines.

1. Be sensitive to the interplay between the various aspects of language on the fluency behavior of the child. Variations in the syntactic-semantic structure in a child's utterance can have a significant impact on the types and extent of the disfluencies the child exhibits.

2. Be mindful of the child's individual threshold of tolerance for linguistic complexity. Thresholds vary from child to child and, at least during therapy for stuttering, one must be careful not to overstretch the child's linguistic limits, which might result in a greater degree of disfluencies.

3. Be mindful of the influence of pragmatic contexts on the child's stuttering. Some communication situations carry greater stress for the child than others. Moreover, the particular pragmatic intention of a communication act can also have profound influence on the child's stuttering. The contexts of utterances and their influence on a child's subsequent communication, including the fluency of his speech, are of particular interest in the current trend of using language samples as a primary means of communication assessment.

4. If using high structured, standardized tests for language assessment,

be cognizant of the author's perspective on language and the validity and reliability of the test.

5. Be mindful of individual differences in the kinds of patterns of fluency and language behaviors exhibited across children.

6. Despite the emphasis of this chapter on psycholinguistic variables, the reader is encouraged to consider the contributions to fluency of various psychosocial and physiological factors that are likely to co-occur with psycholinguistic variables. For example, production of a longer, more complex sentence may also require a more sustained and complex level of motor coordination.

REFERENCES

Andrews, G., and Harris, M. 1964. The Syndrome of Stuttering. Clinics in Developmental Medicine, no. 17. Spastics Society Medical Education and Information Unit in association with William Heinemann Medical Books, London.

Bellak, L., and Bellak, S. 1959. Children's Apperception Test. 3rd Ed. C.P.S., New York.

Bernstein, N. 1981. Are there constraints on childhood disfluency? J. Fluency Disord. 6:341–350.

Berry, M. 1938. Developmental history of stuttering children. J. Pediatr. 12:209–217.

Berryman, J., and Kools, J. 1975. Disfluency of nonstuttering children in relation to specific measures of language, reading, and mental maturity. J. Fluency Disord. 1:18–24.

Bjerkan, B. 1980. Word fragmentations and repetitions in the spontaneous speech of 2–6-year-old children. J. Fluency Disord. 5:137–148.

Blood, G., and Seider, R. 1981. The concomitant problems of young stutterers. J. Speech Hear. Disord. 46:31–33.

Bloodstein, O. 1974. The rules of early stuttering. J. Speech Hear. Disord. 39:379–394.

Bloodstein, O. 1981. A Handbook on Stuttering. 3rd Ed. National Easter Seal Society, Chicago.

Bloodstein, O., and Gantwerk, B. 1967. Grammatical function in relation to stuttering in young children. J. Speech Hear. Res. 10:786–789.

Bloodstein, O., and Grossman, M. 1981. Early stutterings: Some aspects of their form and distribution. J. Speech Hear. Res. 24:298–302.

Bloom, L. 1967. A comment on Lee's "Developmental Sentence Types": A method for comparing normal and deviant syntactic development. J. Speech Hear. Disord. 32:294–296.

Bloom, L. 1970. Language Development: Form and Function in Emerging Grammars. MIT Press, Cambridge, Mass.

Bloom, L., and Lahey, M. 1978. Language Development and Language Disorders. John Wiley & Sons, New York.

Boysen, A., and Cullinan, W. 1971. Object-naming latency in stuttering and nonstuttering children. J. Speech Hear. Res. 14:728–738.

Bransford, J., and McCarrell, M. 1972. Some thoughts about understanding what it means to comprehend. Paper presented at the Conference on Cognition and Symbolic Functions, Pennsylvania State University, University Park.

Brown, R. 1973. A First Language: The Early Stages. Harvard University Press, Cambridge, Mass.

Brown, S. 1937. The influence of grammatical function on the incidence of stuttering. J. Speech Disord. 2:207–215.

Brown, S. 1938. Stuttering with relation to word accent and word position. J. Abnorm. Social Psychol. 33:112–120.

Brown, S. 1945. The loci of stutterings in the speech sequence. J. Speech Disord. 10:181–192.

Carrow, E. 1973. Test for Auditory Comprehension of Language. Teaching Resources Corporation, Boston.

Carrow, E. 1974. Carrow Elicited Language Inventory. Learning Concepts, Austin, Tex.

Cecconi, C., Hood, S., and Tucker, R. 1977. Influence of reading level difficulty on the disfluencies of normal children. J. Speech Hear. Res. 20:463–474.

Chomsky, N. 1957. Syntactic Structures. Mouten, the Hague, the Netherlands.

Chomsky, N. 1959. Review of Skinner's *Verbal Behavior*. Language. 35:26–58.

Colburn, N., and Mysak, E. 1982. Developmental disfluency and emerging grammar. II. Co-occurrence of disfluency with specified semantic-syntactic structures. J. Speech Hear. Res. 25:421–427.

Davis, D. 1939. The relation of repetitions in the speech of young children to certain measures of language maturity and situational factors. Part I. J. Speech Disord. 4:303–318.

Davis, D. 1940. The relation of repetitions in the speech of young children to certain measures of language maturity and situational factors. Parts II and III. J. Speech Disord. 5:235–246.

Dore, J. 1975. Holophrases, speech acts, and language universals. J. Child Lang. 2:21–40.

Dunn, L. 1965. Peabody Picture Vocabulary Test. American Guidance Service, Circle Pines, Minn.

Dunn, L. 1981. Peabody Picture Vocabulary Test—Revised. American Guidance Service, Circle Pines, Minn.

Eisenson, J. 1958. A perseverative theory of stuttering. In: J. Eisenson (ed.), Stuttering: A Symposium, pp. 223–271. Harper & Row, New York.

Eisenson, J. 1975. Stuttering as perseverative behavior. In: J. Eisenson (ed.), Stuttering: A Second Symposium, pp. 401–452. Harper & Row, New York.

Eisenson, J., and Horowitz, E. 1945. The influence of propositionality on stuttering. J. Speech Disord. 10:193–197.

Gordon, P. 1982. The effects of syntactic complexity on the occurrence of disfluencies in five year old children. Unpublished doctoral dissertation, University of Tennessee, Knoxville.

Hall, P. 1977. The occurrence of disfluency in language-disordered school-age children. J. Speech Hearing Disord. 42:364–369.

Halliday, M. 1974. A sociosemiotic perspective on language development. Bull. School Orient. Afr. Stud. 37:60–81.

Haynes, W., and Hood, S. 1977. An investigation of linguistic and fluency variables in nonstuttering children from discrete chronological age groups. J. Fluency Disord. 2:57–74.

Haynes, W., and Hood, S. 1978. Disfluency changes in children as a function of the systematic modification of linguistic complexity. J. Commun. Disord. 11:79–93.

Hegde, M. 1981. Fluency and dysfluencies as language production phenomena. A.S.H.A. 23(abstr.):802.

Helmreich, H., and Bloodstein, O. 1973. The grammatical factor in childhood disfluency in relation to the continuity hypothesis. J. Speech Hear. Res. 16:731–738.

Jakobovits, L. 1966. Utilization of semantic satiation in stuttering: A theoretical analysis. J. Speech Hear. Disord. 31:105–114.

Johnson, W. 1955. A study of the onset and development of stuttering. In W. Johnson and R. Leutenegger (eds.), Stuttering in Children and Adults, pp. 37–73. University of Minnesota Press, Minneapolis.

Johnson, W., and Associates. 1959. The Onset of Stuttering. University of Minnesota Press, Minneapolis.

Johnson, W., and Leutenegger, R. (eds.). 1955. Stuttering in Children and Adults. University of Minnesota Press, Minneapolis.

Kirk, S., McCarthy, J., and Kirk, W. 1968. The Illinois Tests of Psycholinguistic Abilities. Rev. Ed. University of Illinois Press, Urbana.

Kline, M., and Starkweather, C. 1979. Receptive and expressive language performance in young stutterers. A.S.H.A. 21(abstr.):797.

Lee, L. 1966. Developmental sentence types: A method for comparing normal and deviant syntactic development. J. Speech Hear. Disord. 31:311–330.

Lee, L. 1971. Northwestern Syntax Screening Test. Northwestern University Press, Evanston, Ill.

Manning, W., and Riensche, L. 1976. Auditory assembly abilities of stuttering and nonstuttering children. J. Speech Hear. Res. 19:777–783.

McCarthy, D. 1930. The Language Development of the Preschool Child. Institute of Child Welfare Monograph Series, no. 4, pp. 492–630. University of Minnesota Press, Minneapolis.

McCarthy, D. 1954. Language development in children. In: L. Carmichael (ed.), Manual of Child Psychology. John Wiley & Sons, New York.

Merits-Patterson, R., and Reed, C. 1981. Disfluencies in the speech of language-delayed children. J. Speech Hear. Res. 24:55–58.

Metraux, R. 1950. Speech profiles of the pre-school child 18–54 months. J. Speech Disord. 15:37–53.

Miller, J., and Yoder, D. 1972. A syntax teaching program. In: J. McLean, D. Yoder, and R. Schiefelbusch (eds.), Language Intervention with the Retarded, pp. 191–211. University Park Press, Baltimore.

Morley, M. 1967. The Development and Disorders of Speech in Childhood. 2nd Ed. Williams & Wilkins Company, Baltimore.

Muma, J. 1971. Syntax of preschool fluent and disfluent speech: A transformational analysis. J. Speech Hear. Res. 14:428–441.

Murray, H., and Reed, C. 1977. Language abilities of preschool stuttering children. J. Fluency Disord. 2:171–176.

Pearl, S., and Bernthal, J. 1980. The effect of grammatical complexity upon disfluency behavior of nonstuttering preschool children. J. Fluency Disord. 5:55–68.

Perozzi, J. 1970. Phonetic skill (sound-mindedness) of stuttering children. J. Commun. Disord. 3:207–210.

Perozzi, J., and Kunze, L. 1969. Language abilities of stuttering children. Fol. Phoniatr. 21:386–392.

Prutting, C. 1979. Process: The action of moving forward progressively from one point to another on the way to completion. J. Speech Hear. Disord. 44:3–30.

Prutting, C. 1982. Pragmatics as social competence. J. Speech Hearing Disord. 47:123–134.

Prutting, C., Gallagher, T., and Mulac, A. 1975. The expressive portion of the NSST compared to a spontaneous language sample. J. Speech Hear. Disord. 40:40–49.

Schlesinger, I. 1974. Relational concepts underlying language. In: R. Schiefelbusch and L. Lloyd (eds.), Language Perspectives—Acquisition, Retardation and Interventions, pp. 129–151. University Park Press, Baltimore.

Shriberg, L., and Kwiatkowski, J. 1982. Phonological disorders. I: A diagnostic classification system. J. Speech Hear. Disord. 47:226–241.

Sichel, R. 1973. Initial phoneme in relation to disfluency in the spontaneous speech of nonstuttering preschool children. Unpublished master's thesis, Brooklyn College, New York.

Siegel, G. 1979. Appraisal of language development. In: F. Darley (ed.), Evaluation of Appraisal Techniques in Speech and Language Pathology, pp. 1–3. Addison-Wesley Publishing Company, Reading, Mass.

Silverman, E.-M. 1972a. Generality of disfluency data collected from preschoolers. J. Speech Hear. Res. 15:84–92.

Silverman, E.-M. 1972b. Preschoolers' speech disfluency: Single syllable word repetition. Percep. Motor Skills. 35:1002.

Silverman, E.-M. 1972c. Syntactic complexity of preschoolers' egocentric and socialized speech. Percep. Motor Skills. 35:247–249.

Silverman, E.-M. 1973a. Clustering: A characteristic of preschoolers' disfluency. J. Speech Hear. Res. 16:578–583.

Silverman, E.-M. 1973b. The influence of preschoolers' speech usage on their disfluency frequency. J. Speech Hear. Res. 16:474–481.

Silverman, E.-M. 1974. Word position and grammatical function in relation to preschoolers' speech disfluency. Percep. Motor Skills. 39:267–272.

Silverman, E.-M. 1975. Effect of selected word attributes on preschoolers' speech disfluency: Initial phoneme and length. J. Speech Hear. Res. 18:430–434.

Silverman, E.-M., and Williams, D. 1967. A comparison of stuttering and nonstuttering children in terms of five measures of oral language development. J. Commun. Disord. 1:305–309.

Silverman, F., and Williams, D. 1973. Use of revision by elementary-school stutterers and nonstutterers during oral reading. J. Speech Hear. Res. 16:584–585.

Soderberg, G. 1967. Linguistic factors in stuttering. J. Speech Hear. Res. 10:801–810.

Starkweather, C. 1980. Speech fluency and its development in normal children. In: N. Lass (ed.), Speech and Language: Advances in Basic Research and Practice, pp. 143–200, Vol. 4. Academic Press, New York.

Stocker, B. 1980. Stocker Probe Technique: For Diagnosis and Treatment of Stuttering in Young Children. Modern Education Corporation, Tulsa.

Stocker, B., and Parker, E. 1977. The relationship between auditory recall and disfluency in young stutterers. J. Fluency Disord. 2:177–187.

Taylor, I. 1966. What words are stuttered? Psychol. Bull. 65:233–242.

Templin, M. 1957. Certain Language Skills in Children. University of Minnesota Press, Minneapolis.

Tiffany, W. 1963. Sound mindedness: Studies in the measurement of "phonetic ability." West. Speech. 27:5–15.

Van Riper, C. 1982. The Nature of Stuttering. 2nd Ed. Prentice-Hall, Englewood Cliffs, N.J.

Vellutino, F., and Shub, M. 1982. Assessment of disorders in formal school language: disorders in reading. In: K. Butler (ed.) and R. Calfee (issue ed.), Topics in Language Disorders, pp. 20–33, Vol. 2. Aspen Systems Corporation, Gaithersburg, Md.

Wall, M. 1980. A comparison of syntax in young stutterers and nonstutterers. J. Fluency Disord. 5:345–352.

Wall, M., Starkweather, C., and Cairns, H. 1981. Syntactic influences on stuttering in young children stutterers. J. Fluency Disord. 6:283–298.

Westby, C. 1979. Language performance of stuttering and nonstuttering children. J. Commun. Disord. 12:133–145.

Williams, A., and Marks, C. 1972. A comparative analysis of the ITPA and PPVT performance of young stutterers. J. Speech Hear. Res. 15:323–329.

Williams, D., and Silverman, F. 1968. Note concerning articulation of school-age stutterers. Percept. Motor Skills. 27:713–714.

Williams, D., Silverman, F., and Kools, J. 1969. Disfluency behavior of elementary-school stutterers and nonstutterers: Loci of instances of disfluency. J. Speech Hear. Res. 12:308–318.

Wingate, M. 1967. Slurvian skill of stutterers. J. Speech Hear. Res. 10:844–848.

Wingate, M. 1976. Stuttering: Theory and Treatment. John Wiley & Sons, New York.

Wingate, M. 1977. The immediate source of stuttering: An integration of evidence. J. Commun. Disord. 10:45–51.

Wingate, M. 1979. The loci of stuttering: Grammar or prosody? Commun. Disord. 12:283–290.

5
The Physiology of Childhood Stuttering

Physiological maturation for speech production occurs during the language-learning years when stuttering so frequently begins. The language and speech systems are more easily considered and discussed separately, yet they function as an intergrated and harmonious unit in most speakers. Having examined the linguistic aspects of early fluency, nonfluency, and stuttering in Chapter 4, we now focus on the physiological aspects of speech production in young children, namely, the early development of the speech production mechanism, its effect on early speech production, and the maturely functioning mechanism. In addition, we present studies examining the speech production of child stutterers and attempt to integrate the current but limited information into theoretical and clinical considerations.

MATURATION OF THE SPEECH MECHANISM

Early Development

Major anatomical and physiological alterations in the speech production system take place during the first few years of life; these changes put the system in a state of maturational flux during that time. This is in marked contrast to the smoothly coordinated system underlying mature speech production.

In the respiratory system, mature breathing patterns are established at about 7 years of age. By that time the lungs have reached full, or almost full, growth. The rib cage enclosing the lungs has also undergone changes, in that the ribs become increasingly angled after age 2, and by age 7 the rib cage is similar to that in adults (Kahane, 1982). Physiological alterations occur with the anatomical changes, and the high rate of 60 to 70 breaths per minute of infancy reduces over time to 16 to 18 breaths per minute in the adult. In addition, the diaphragmatic breathing of the infant changes to a mixed pattern of diaphragmatic and thoracic breathing at about 6 months of age, and remains until 7 years, when thoracic movements predominate (Peiper, 1963). These observations apply to quiet respiration; few data are available on respiratory patterns of young children during speech production.

Moving superiorly from the respiratory system, the infant's vocal tract differs from the mature vocal tract in that the larynx is positioned higher, close to the oral cavity (Negus, 1949). This allows respiratory access to the nasal passages during suckling. The epiglottis is also more superiorly placed, its tip close to the soft palate, and the tongue is forward in the mouth. The resulting configuration is of a single, almost horizontal tube, rather than the two-tube, elbow-shaped vocal tract of the adult. Consequently, however, the infant has little pharyngeal space; this area develops along with the more mature vocal tract. In addition, the infant has very little vertical laryngeal mobility because of the close proximity of the thyroid cartilage and the hyoid bone.

By age 2, the shape of the supraglottal tract is more like that of the adult, although further fine anatomical adjustments occur. The larynx, for example, initially located at a level between the first and second cervical vertebrae, gradually descends, reaching the level of the sixth cervical vertebra by adulthood. Kahane (1982) pointed out that the larynx grows rapidly during the first 3 years of life, and then slowly until puberty, when another growth spurt occurs. At that time, the rapid growth of the male vocal folds is reflected in pitch changes, a good example of poorly controlled phonation resulting from anatomical growth and a subsequent alteration in physiology. That is, because of rapid growth, the vocal folds are unable to vibrate with their customary synchrony; the result is fluctuating, uncontrolled pitch changes.

The tongue, which roughly doubles in size from infancy to adulthood, is positioned more posteriorly and inferiorly by age 4, as the larynx descends. Soft palate growth occurs largely during the child's first 2 years then it grows more gradually until about 4 years, and thereafter increases somewhat in length until 18 years of age (Subtelny, 1957). Add to these continuing adjustments the development of jaw movement, and to a lesser extent, facial muscle activity—already fairly well developed in infancy.

By the time the child is 5 years old, the upper vocal tract has become the bent, two-tube mechanism of the mature speaker, with all spatial relationships in order. The early language and speech falterings of the young child are more easly understood when viewed in the context of developing linguistic and physiological systems—the systems apparently developing simultaneously and synergistically.

Maturational Effects on Speech Production

Increasing control of the speech production mechanism is reflected in maturing speech production. In addition to longitudinal work that delineates developing articulatory and phonological skills (Sander, 1972), more microscopic articulatory research has focused on the finely tuned coordination required for speech. Kent (1976) summarized a good deal of research in this area, pointing out that several aspects of speech and voice production are occurring simultaneously. Voice onset time (VOT) is an example of an element of articulation that has been studied developmentally (see Chapter 2 for definition and further discussion).

For the first 3 years of life, VOT is not divided into one onset time for voiced consonants and another onset time for voiceless consonants—forming a bimodal distribution—as is the case with adult VOT. Rather, during early childhood, voiced and voiceless consonants have similar VOT's. The more mature VOT develops gradually and is not achieved until about 8 years of age. Thus the development of speech physiology underlies the development of the finer laryngeal adjustments, and their coordination with the articulators, that are required for adult VOT. Physiological maturation for speech occurs within the time span that stuttering most often develops. Moreover, it is possible that poorly coordinated speech attempts of some children may be further burdened by the concurrently developing linguistic demands of the system. The result could be an overburdened speech and language output system.

The Mature Mechanism

Basic to the trend in physiological research of the stutterer's speech production mechanism is knowledge of ways in which events in the larynx influence phonation and the synergistic interaction of all components of the speech production mechanism. It is known, for example, that phonation depends on a delicate balance of muscular and nonmuscular forces at the level of the vocal folds. These forces need to be well timed, well sequenced, and well coordinated.

Throughout speech and voice production in running speech there is continuous reciprocity between the adductor (lateral cricoarytenoid, interarytenoid), the abductor (posterior cricoarytenoid), and the tensor (vocalis, cricothyroid) muscles of the larynx. This reciprocal muscle action, as well as the aerodynamic events that originate in the subglottal area, are necessary for appropriate onset and maintenance of phonation, and for the occurrence of voiced and voiceless segments of sounds in running speech. Any interruption or lack of coordination in this complex synergistic arrangement may result in a poorly regulated phonatory attempt.

The sound from the glottis is altered by the resonating cavities of the supraglottal tract and is shaped into intelligible speech by the articulators. The final, articulated string of words is organized into chunks, or clauses, which give syntactic definition to the utterance. Underlying the syntactic pattern of clause units is respiration for speech, and for fluent speech, respiration usually occurs at clause boundaries. Fodor, Bever, and Garret (1974) noted that ". . . the coincidence of breathing with syntactically defined units reflects true integration of respiration patterns with sentence planning activities" (p. 425).

The end product to which the child aspires, therefore, is complex and dynamic. The child may experience breakdown in a component part or parts, altering the synergy of the system; or the parts may be difficult to coordinate, again altering the synergy required for fluent speech.

STUDIES OF SPEECH PRODUCTION

In this section we examine studies that have been carried out on childhood stutterers. In some areas—particularly in respiration—the studies are sparse in comparison with the existing adult research. The topics covered are respiration, voice onset time, voice reaction and initiation times, the voicing feature, distinctive features, coarticulation, and consonants versus vowels.

Respiration

As stated in Chapter 2, breathing anomalies have usually been considered to be secondary to the original stuttering condition. Such conclusions were drawn from data of studies on adult stutterers. If breathing aberrations were detected in young stutterers at the onset of stuttering—in a 3-year-old child, for instance—we would be justified in attributing more importance to respiratory difficulties in relation to stuttering. Children's respiratory patterns are not mature until about 7 years of age, however, and so comparisons between groups are difficult. If the norm is quite variable, how variable would aberrant patterns need to be?

Steer (1937) discerned the difficulties of this research when, using pneumographs placed around the thorax and abdomen of each subject, he examined the respiratory patterns during speech of 30 stutterers and 20 nonstutterers. The experimental group age range was 3 to 6 years and the control group ranged in age from 3 to 5 years. Steer found seven breathing patterns that were exhibited by both groups; some patterns were shown more by the stutterers, and some more by the nonstutterers. The stutterers were more likely to speak on inhalation, to show a lack of movement of either the thorax or the abdomen, to have the abdomen and thorax moving in different patterns simultaneously, and to show unequal, successive respiratory wave forms. The nonstutterers more frequently showed unusually long duration of inhalation and exhalation, and more frequently interrupted their exhalation by inhaling. Both groups demonstrated oppositional movements of abdomen and thorax fairly evenly. Steer noted that 60% of the stutterers had four or more of the seven symptoms, and 55% of the nonstutterers had four or more symptoms.

Looking at Steer's work more closely, some of the comparisons showed substantial contrasts, whereas others did not. For example, 70% of the nonstutterers had "unusually long duration of inspiration and expiration," but this description applied to only 26.6% of the stutterers. (One must wonder whether "long duration" is not, perhaps, the norm.) Of the stutterers, 90% spoke on inhalation, as opposed to 45% of the nonstutterers. For "general equality in successive wave forms," the difference between the two groups was less marked—46.7% of the stutterers and 35% of the nonstutterers.

This pioneering work does not appear to have been replicated, although it suggests, in some areas, important differences between the two groups of children. It also demonstrates, however, that many youngsters—stutterers or not—are experiencing "anomalies" of a developing respiratory system. Perhaps one reason for the failure to pursue this type of research is that, for the most part, the work on older stutterers reflected a normally functioning respiratory system at rest, and further research was not deemed necessary. In addition, such research is particularly difficult with children, who do not take kindly to sitting still for long periods of time attached to instrumentation.

Voice Onset Time

The time between the release of the articulators and the onset of voicing (voice onset time, VOT) and the time between the end of voicing and articulatory movement for the following consonant (voice termination time, VTT) may be measured on a spectrogram. Because this process is not invasive, it is appropriate for use with young children. Predictably, however, it has been used more frequently on adults than on children.

Agnello, Wingate, and Wendell (1974) examined VOT and VTT in the fluent syllables of 12 child stutterers aged 5 to 7 years. Twelve normally fluent children and 12 adult stutterers acted as controls. The experimental group exhibited longer VOT's than the control group of children, and longer VOT's and VTT's than the adult controls. The adult stutterers, in turn, showed longer VOT's and VTT's than their adult controls. The VOT data on adult stutterers were confirmed by Hillman and Gilbert (1977), who studied VOT in perceptually fluent syllables taken from the connected speech of 10 subjects, but were not confirmed by Metz, Conture, and Caruso (1979) in a study of only 5 subjects.

The above-mentioned findings suggest that the mistimings found in the adult stutterers' speech production may have existed quite early in life. As in respiration, if the mistimings are present from the onset of stuttering a physiological component to the onset can be posited. There have been no reports on young children who have been examined close to the time of the onset of the condition. And because we know that VOT is not as stable in the youngster as it is in the mature speaker, a sizable data base is advisable before we speculate about etiology. It is also possible that the mistimings in adult stutterers have in some way resulted from the physical tension of stuttering, or they may represent "minimal" stuttering (Bloodstein, 1981) or "subacoustic" stuttering (Starkweather, 1982).

Voice Reaction and Initiation Times

As in the adult studies, researchers have been interested in whether child stutterers are capable of reacting quickly motorically on a number of levels. Studies have focused on finger reaction time (FRT) as well as voice reaction time (VRT) or voice initiation time (VIT). More than one of these variables are studied because of an interest in whether stuttering moments are the result of an aberrant voice/speech production mechanism, or whether they are part of a more widespread motor disturbance.

Luper and Cross (1978) and Cross and Luper (1979) found that childhood stutterers had longer FRT's and VRT's than their matched controls. For the FRT study the subjects were in three groups of nine at age levels of 5 years, 9 years, and adult. The subjects pressed a telegraph key as quickly as possible upon hearing a 1,000 Hz, 80 dB tone onset, and released it at tone offset. The mean FRT for stutterers *and* nonstutterers decreased as the subjects increased in age, with the greatest change occurring between 5 and 9 years. As a group, the stutterers exhibited significantly longer FRT's than nonstutterers, and intrasubject variability was greater for the stutterers than for the nonstutterers.

For the VRT study, Cross and Luper (1979) used the three groups of 5-year-olds, 9-year-olds, and adult stutterers matched to nonstutterers. The subjects phonated /ʌ/ as quickly as possible upon hearing a 1,000-Hz tone. Of the stutterers, 5-year-olds had the longest VRT's with a mean of 562 msec; 9-year-olds means were shorter, at 351 msec, and adults had the shortest VRT, with a mean of 300 msec. Considering the stutterers and nonstutterers together, the 5-year-old VRT differed significantly from the 9-year-old VRT, and from the adult VRT, with no difference between the 9-year-olds and adults.

Luper and Cross (1978) and Cross and Luper (1979) consider that neuromuscular maturation underlies the improved FRT and VRT over time in both stutterers and nonstutterers. Because longer VRT has been found almost consistently in adult stutterers when compared with nonstutterers (see, e.g., Adams and Hayden, 1976; Cross, Shadden, and Luper, 1979; Lewis, Ingham, and Gervens, 1979; Reich, Till, and Goldsmith, 1981; Starkweather, Hirschman, and Tannenbaum, 1976), Cross and Luper seem to be justified in theorizing that the early latent VRT's might contribute to the onset of fluency difficulties, rather than resulting from them or being an integral part of them, as has been suggested.

Further reaction time research on young stutterers has not necessarily supported the results above, but variables such as age of subjects and severity of stuttering differ so greatly that comparisons are difficult. In all the following studies a stimulus tone was used to elicit reactions from the subjects. Cullinan and Springer (1980) measured VIT and voice termination time (VTT) in 20 stutterers aged 5.8 to 11.7 years. Eleven of the children had language, learning, and speech difficulties in addition to stuttering. As a group, the stutterers had significantly longer VIT and VTT measures than the nonstutterers. However, in contrast to Cross and Luper's study, the younger subjects (under 8 years of age) had VIT—and VTT—scores that did not differ from those of the control group, whereas the scores of children over 8 years differed significantly on both measures. These findings suggest that stutterers' difficulties in managing the vocal mechanism may emerge over time, in direct contrast to the conclusions from Cross and Luper's study. The 11 stutterers who had language, learning, and speech difficulties (5 of whom were under 8 years) exhibited significantly longer VIT's and VTT's than the control group, suggesting a very broadly based linguistic deficit.

In addition to linguistic variables, Cullinan and Springer considered severity of stuttering, and found that severity did not affect their results. That is, when the 11 mild to moderate stutterers were grouped, and the 9 moderate to severe stutterers were grouped, differences between the groups on the two measures were not significant. Starkweather (1982, p. 21) points out, however, that with two-thirds of the comparisons in the expected direction (12 of 18 comparisons showed that milder stutterers had faster reaction times), a difference in reaction time due to severity should not be ruled out. Cullinan and Springer's attempts to group their subjects according to linguistic deficits and severity of stuttering are encouraging, because the heterogeneity of stutterers is frequently ignored in stuttering research (see Watson and Alfonso (1982, 1983) for observed influences of stuttering severity on reaction time in adult stutterers).

In a further study of VIT and VTT, Murphy and Baumgartner (1981), like Cullinan and Springer, found no differences between reaction times of young stutterers (average age 5 years 8 months) and nonstutterers. There were widely disparate rates of stuttering among the subjects of this study. Controlling for rate of stuttering by using moderate to severe stutterers, Reich and Till (1981) tested FRT as well as voice and speech reaction times on 13 stutterers with an average age of 10.6 years. The tasks were button pressing, inspiratory phonation, expiratory throat clearing, the productions of /ʌ/ and the word /ʌpɚ/. The mean reaction times of the stutterers were significantly longer than those of the nonstutterers for throat clearing and the initiation of /ʌpɚ/. According to these results, it was more difficult for the children to initiate voice for the word /ʌpɚ/ than for the vowel /ʌ/, which was not delayed. This makes sense in that the demands for voicing and motor planning for a word should be more complex than for a vowel, but subjects of roughly equivalent age—Cullinan and Springer's older children—exhibited longer VIT's than controls for a vowel sound. The nonphonatory task of throat clearing, which was also delayed, presumably implies a slow response of the stutterers' larynges generally, regardless of whether phonation is involved. Other measures did not differ between the two groups.

The reaction time studies are difficult to compare because of the differences in methodology. The results obtained by Cross and Luper were not supported by the two studies that also contained younger children (Cullinan and Springer, 1980; Murphy and Baumgartner, 1981) but this may have been because of methodological differences. The work of Cross and Luper and Luper and Cross demonstrating comparisons in reaction time at different age levels is appealing in the logic of the studies, but the severity of the subjects' stuttering is unknown. The suggestion that FRT and VRT may become shorter and more adult-like over time is also appealing because it fits into a plausible theory of maturation for both stutterers and nonstutterers, in which the stutterers are simply less proficient than their fluent counterparts. Further studies with groups of children at the various age levels are desirable to clarify the role of reaction time in childhood stuttering.

The Voicing Feature

Further speech production research has sought information on whether the larynx as an articulator influences the site and rate of stuttering. Attempts to associate stuttering with laryngeal adjustments for voiced and voiceless sounds have met with limited success. Adams and Reis (1971) examined the location of stuttering in relation to the initiation of voice in a speech segment taken from oral reading by adult stutterers. In one paragraph all sounds were voiced, requiring fewer laryngeal adjustments than the second paragraph, which contained a combination of voiced and voiceless sounds. The authors found significantly less stuttering in the all-voiced passage than in the combined passage and speculated that "spasmic glottal closures" may account for stuttering that occurs in such locations.

Replicating their study, Adams and Reis (1974) found that the all-voiced material did not produce significantly less stuttering than the combined passage. In both studies, however, adaptation (the tendency for stuttering to decrease with successive readings of the same passage) was significantly higher in the combined passage than in the all-voiced passage.

Wall, Starkweather, and Cairns (1981) and Wall, Starkweather, and Harris (1981), studying the spontaneous speech of nine preschool stutterers, did not find that voiced-voiceless transitions influenced the rate of stuttering. They did find that the initiation of voice at the onset of a sentence or clause, or after any kind of pause, was an extremely powerful factor in increasing the rate of stuttering. Stuttering occurred with an average frequency of 19% where word initiation followed a clause or sentence boundary, or a pause of some kind within an utterance. Stuttering was fairly evenly distributed at these locations, whether the first sound of the word was voiced or voiceless. Stuttering occurred with an average frequency of only 4%, however, at other locations in utterances where a variety of voiced-voiceless transitions were examined.

Still focusing on the work by Adams and Reis, two attempts were made to replicate on school-aged children the findings of these authors. Using a similar paradigm, McGee, Hutchinson, and Deputy (1981) asked stutterers from grades 3 through 7 to read a passage containing all-voiced sounds and one containing a normal distribution of voiced and voiceless sounds. There was no significant difference in the rate of adaptation. Also, Runyon and Bonifant (1981), whose subjects had an average age of 9 years 9 months, found no difference in the rate of stuttering between two similarly constructed passages.

The presence or absence of the voicing feature does not seem to affect the occurrence of stuttering. The initiation of voice/speech from silence, whether the first sound of the word is voiced or voiceless, however, is a fairly powerful predictor of stuttering in preschool children. This finding, of course, may reflect a number of converging variables that underlie spoken utterances—sentence planning and organization may be taking place at the beginning of a sentence or clause. This activity must be coordinated with respiration for speech, and all activities must be coordinated with the initiation of phonation and speech.

Distinctive Features

Wall and Pfeuffer (1978) performed a distinctive feature analysis of spontaneous speech samples of 11 stutterers, aged 4 and 5 years. They found that the most frequently occurring features in the initial sound of a stuttered word were (+tense), (+low), (+continuant), (+vocalic), whereas for the second part of the word the features were (+consonantal) and (+nasal). Because these features describe the first two sounds of the word "and," with which young children frequently begin their clauses, the overlap of articulatory and semantic-syntactic influences on stuttering is apparent. As stutterers mature, they begin their clauses with a greater variety of words, including words beginning with consonants. This may account for the change in rate of stuttering on consonants versus vowels in the older stutterer.

Consonants versus Vowels

Adults have consistently exhibited high rates of stuttering on words beginning with consonants as opposed to words beginning with vowels (Brown,

1945; Hejna, 1955; Taylor, 1966). Two recent studies suggest that this dichotomy is irrelevant to preschool stutterers. Bloodstein and Grossman (1981) reported on five children aged 3 years, 10 months to 5 years, 7 months who, as a group, did not stutter more on consonant-initiated words than on vowel-initiated words, although that tendency existed for the oldest child in the group. Supportive data were reported by Wall, Stark-weather, and Harris (1981) with regard to nine stutterers aged 4 to 6 years, 6 months. Williams, Silverman, and Kools (1969) found a tendency toward consonant-related stuttering in 5- to 13-year-olds. This suggests a shift over time in the stuttered sounds—from no tendency in the preschoolers, to a tendency in the older children, to a significant difference in the rate of stuttering on consonants versus vowels in the older stutterer. In view of previous linguistic findings, however, the shift from vowel stuttering to consonant stuttering seems to be due primarily to language maturation rather than to a physiologically based shift.

Coarticulation

Another way to examine the synchrony and timing of articulatory events is through observation of how speech sounds interlock and overlap with each other, or how we coarticulate. Coarticulation is impaired when the stutterer blocks, as in bu—bu—bu—baby, or ba—ba—ba—baby, or ba—(phona-tory arrest or pitch glide)—aby. Speakers usually achieve transitions be-tween sounds and overlapping articulatory movements easily and fluidly; stutterers' blocks are an example of extreme difficulty in this normal process.

Stromsta (1965) addressed the issue of the transition in stuttered speech when he examined spectrograms of children reported to stutter. The acoustic cues of the spectrograms were evaluated with regard to those of the youngsters who became persistent stutterers during the next 10 years. The children who became persistent stutterers are said to have exhibited two characteristic patterns: one that reflected abrupt phonatory stoppages, and a lack of transitional formants related to the vowels of syllabic repeti-tions. Coarticulation is presumed to have been difficult for these children in light of the inadequate transitional movement. The children who did not exhibit abrupt phonatory stoppages and poor coarticulation are reported to have spontaneously developed normal speech. This work is of interest because it suggests that the phonatory aberrations and coarticulatory diffi-culties are present early in life, and by the relatively simple method of making spectrograms, we may differentially diagnose the child who is destined to become a confirmed stutter. In spite of the powerful implica-tions of this report, no longitudinal research has been carried out to con-firm or invalidate Stromsta's observations.

In a study related to the timing of segments of formant transitions and steady state duration, Healey (1981) studied spectrograms of utterances produced by 10 mild stutterers (average age 9.7 years) and 10 matched controls. All subjects produced the sentence "Pass the sauce to me," from which the analyses were made. In marking transitions and steady state subsegments, Healey defined 11 landmarks of the utterance /əsɔs/, from "the sauce." For the initial segments, no significant differences were found in the timing between the stutterers and controls. Significant differences were found between the two groups for two final transitional subsegments of onset and offset of frication, in that the times of the stutterers were longer for two subsegments than the times of the controls. The author suggested that these data in part support a study by Starkweather and Myers (1979) in which intervocalic portions of /əsʌ/—taken from *the sunlight*—were examined. Starkweather and Myers's subjects (age range 10 to 31 years) also had slower transitional subsegments than fluent speakers. These transitional data may also be viewed in terms of the timing difficulties of stutterers raised previously in this chapter and in Chapter 2.

Further transitional data, on adults, are offered by Zimmermann (1980) who examined fluent CVC utterances of stutterers through cineradiography. He found longer transition times and longer steady state vowels in stutterers than in nonstutterers. By contrast, Hand and Luper (1980), using plosives in CVC units (as did Zimmermann), found shorter transition times for adult stutterers.

Transitional data in both child and adult populations are limited, and we lack enough information to make an informed judgment as to whether coarticulation in the fluent utterances of stutterers occurs normally in either population.

Conture and his colleagues at Syracuse University are engaged in ongoing research that is pertinent to the above discussion. Zebrowski, Conture, and Cudahy (1983) presented, as part of this large-scale study, findings on the temporal characteristics of speech events for 11 stutterers and matched controls, aged 3 to 7 years. They pointed out that for plosive production of the nonstutterers, there is a systematically varied relation between the duration of aspiration and the duration of the stop gap—the time of the closure of the articulators for the plosive. That is, a longer aspiration is associated with a shorter stop gap. The young stutterers, however, showed little or no relation between the durations of aspiration and the stop gap. It was suggested that "multiple release bursts"—presumably attempts to release the plosive—may be responsible for the increased duration of the stop gap. Although the multiple release bursts are found in fluent children's speech, they are more common in the speech of the stutterers (Caruso, Conture, Cudahy, and Schwartz, 1981).

Conture and his colleagues (personal communication) have also found other timing anomalies. For example, electroglottographic data on, to date, five stutterers and controls, compared derived waveforms of the two groups. When degrees of vocal fold abduction per glottal cycle were analyzed, two aberrant patterns emerged from the stutterers' data: inappropriate adduction during consonant production, and sudden, unpredictable increases in the degree of abduction, most visible in vowel production. Some of these patterns existed in the normal speakers' productions, but again, they were more common in the stutterers' speech.

The work of Conture and his colleagues is still in its embryonic stages, but may well contribute the information needed to determine whether the mistimings generally found in mature stutterers' speech are present in early stuttering. So far this careful work is pointing in the direction of very subtle temporal asynchronies in stuttered speech.

LIMITATIONS OF PHYSIOLOGICAL RESEARCH ON CHILDREN

It takes time and ingenuity to collect data of any kind on young children, and if instrumentation is to be used, the problems are compounded. Electromyography, for instance, which has given us information on the laryngeal muscle activity of the fluent and stuttered speech of stutterers, uses hookwires inserted into the desired muscles. This invasive procedure is unsuitable for children. The fiberscope, which consists primarily of a thin bundle of light-carrying glass filaments, may be inserted nasally and allows a view of the pharyngeal and laryngeal areas during running speech. This instrument has allowed viewing and videotaping of events in the larynx for stutterers, and for clients with other pathologies, but it is also an invasive procedure and has not been used on young stutterers.

An instrument that has already proved useful in the study of stuttering in children is the spectrograph, which analyzes and displays speech signals according to the acoustic characteristics of frequency, intensity, and time. The resulting patterns, which are burned into the smoked paper, correspond to the acoustic cues. The cues for vocalic sounds are the formants, and various other cues exist for the variety of consonants—for example, "noise" patterns for fricatives and "burst" patterns for plosives. Because the speech signal is continually changing and because of the coarticulatory influences of speech sounds on each other, adjacent cues tend to merge. In running speech, transitions (or frequency shifts of the formants) occur as the cues for the vowel merge with the cues for the adjacent sounds. VOT can be detected by examining the cue for voicing in relation to the cue for the release of the articulators.

The glottograph and the laryngograph offer indirect methods of evaluating the waveform emanating from the glottis. Glottography is a process of transillumination, using a photocell to measure the amount of light shining through the glottis. The laryngograph, on the other hand, gives a waveform that reflects the closed phase of the vocal folds. The impedance between the adducted folds is measured through surface electrodes placed on either side of the larynx. Respiratory measures of thoracic and abdominal movements may be made by transducers placed around the pertinent areas of the child's body.

In view of the difficulties of the use of instrumentation on young children, further mention of the work of Conture and his associates is appropriate at this point. Their overall plan includes the collection of respiratory and acoustic information, electroglottographic waveform analysis, and surface EMG recordings of labial muscles (orbicularis oris and depressor labii inferior) used in speech production. Such painstaking work should result in sound information on many aspects of the speech of young nonstutterers, and the fluent and stuttered speech of the stutterers. The timing of physiological events in relation to each other is one focus of this broad study.

THEORETICAL AND CLINICAL CONSIDERATIONS

The persistent finding that adult stutterers have mistimings of laryngeal function and of other areas of the vocal tract during some fluent, as well as stuttered, utterances stimulated speculation regarding a physiological "cause" of stuttering. However, as stated previously in this chapter, some speculate that the "fluent" mistimings are simply very mild forms of stuttering that are not acoustically perceptible, and this is certainly plausible. It is not known whether the fluent mistimings in the vocal tract have developed or whether they were present at the onset of stuttering. If they were present at stuttering onset, perhaps some methods of early detection would clarify the status of the occasional difficult-to-diagnose child.

The physiological work on adults has been indirectly helpful to those working with child stutterers. We are more acutely aware of the physiological concomitants of stuttering that may be present or may develop, and more acutely aware of what we must prevent. Information on the physiological differences occurring immediately prior to moments of stuttering, for example, may help us to design therapy procedures to reduce their effects on stuttering (Myers, 1978). Increasingly, clinicians are finding ways to deal with the motor involvement of some young stutterers (Adams, 1980; Gregory and Hill, 1980; Nelson, 1982; Shine, 1980). At the same time, we require more information on the physiology of stuttering in young children to gain a better understanding of the early stages of the condition, to improve our differential diagnostic techniques, and to continue to refine our therapy for this population.

We have pointed out that the child's language skills are burgeoning along with his neurophysiological maturation for speech production, and that some children have more difficulty than others in coordinating apparently multiple levels of language and speech production. Some children may have particular difficulty with one or more levels of the system: in selection of vocabulary from the lexicon, for example, in structuring a sentence, in coordinating respiration with vocal tract movements, or in achieving a coordinated spatial and temporal integration of articulatory gestures for speech production. Conceivably such children may be candidates for stuttering, insofar as a breakdown at one or more levels could throw the system out of synchronization. To date, the language of the young stutterer has been explored more fully than the physiology of speech production. Further information should be gleaned from acoustic and physiological studies using noninvasive techniques. Such research should include attention to glottal and supraglottal areas and to respiration, and ideally should be coordinated with explorations of the linguistic variables that are suspected to influence the rate and location of stuttering in childhood stutterers.

The physiological research carried out to date has enhanced our knowledge of the stuttering block and of the stutterer's "fluent" speech; it has given direction for further research and therapy and has stimulated more thinking on the physiological nature of stuttering.

REFERENCES

Adams, M. R. 1980. The young stutterer: Diagnosis, treatment and assessment of progress. Semin. Speech Lang. Hear. 1:289–300.

Adams, M. R., and Hayden, P. 1976. The ability of stutterers and nonstutterers to initiate and terminate phonation during production of an isolated vowel. J. Speech Hear. Res. 19:290–296.

Adams, M. R., and Reis, R. 1971. The influence of the onset of phonation on the frequency of stuttering. J. Speech Hear. Res. 14:639–644.

Adams, M. R., and Reis, R. 1974. Influence of the onset of phonation on the frequency of stuttering: A replication and re-evaluation. J. Speech Hear. Res. 17:752–753.

Agnello, J., Wingate, M. E., and Wendell, M. V. 1974. Voice onset and voice termination times of children and adult stutterers. Paper presented at the American Speech and Hearing Association Convention, Las Vegas.

Bloodstein, O. 1981. A Handbook on Stuttering. 3rd Ed. National Easter Seal Society, Chicago.

Bloodstein, O., and Grossman, M. 1981. Early stutterings: Some aspects of their form and distribution. J. Speech Hear. Res. 24:298–302.

Brown, S. F. 1945. The loci of stuttering in the speech sequence. J. Speech Disord. 10:181–192.

Caruso, A. J., Conture, E. G., Cudahy, E. A., and Schwartz, H. D., 1981. Temporal characteristics of young stutterers' fluency. Paper presented at the American Speech-Language-Hearing Convention, Los Angeles.

Cross, D., and Luper, H. 1979. Voice reaction time of stuttering and nonstuttering children and adults. J. Fluency Disord. 4:59–77.

Cross. D. E., Shadden, B. B., and Luper, H. L. 1979. Effects of stimulus presentation on the voice reaction time of adult stutterers and nonstutterers. J. Fluency Disord. 4:45–58.

Cullinan, W. L., and Springer, M. T. 1980. Voice initiation and termination times in stuttering and nonstuttering children. J. Speech Hear. Res. 23:344–360.

Fodor, J. A., Bever, T. G., and Garrett, M. F. 1974. The Psychology of Language. McGraw-Hill Book Company, New York.

Gregory, H. H., and Hill, D. 1980. Stuttering therapy for children. Semin. Speech Lang. Hear. 1:351–363.

Hand, C. R., and Luper, H. L. 1980. Durational characteristics of stutterers' and nonstutterers' fluent speech. Paper presented at the American Speech-Language-Hearing Association Convention, Detroit.

Healey, E. C. 1981. Child stutterers' fluent transition and steady-state subsegment durations. Paper presented at the American Speech-Language-Hearing Association, Los Angeles.

Hejna, R. F. 1955. A study of the loci of stuttering in spontaneous speech. Unpublished doctoral dissertation, Northwestern University, Evanston, Ill.

Hillman, R. E., and Gilbert, H. R. 1977. Voice onset time for voiceless stop consonants in the fluent reading of stutterers and nonstutterers. J. Acoust. Soc. Am. 61:610–611.

Kahane, J. C. 1982. Anatomy and physiology of the organs of the peripheral speech mechanism. In: N. J. Lass, L. V. McReynolds, J. L. Northern, and D. E. Yoder (eds.), Speech, Language, and Hearing, pp. 109–155; Vol. 1, Normal Processes. W. B. Saunders Company, Philadelphia.

Kent, R. 1976. Anatomical and neuromuscular maturation of the speech mechanism: Evidence from acoustic studies. J. Speech Hear. Res. 19:421–447.

Lewis, J. I., Ingham, R. J., and Gervens, A. 1979. Voice initiation and termination times in stutterers and normal speakers. Paper presented at the American Speech and Hearing Association Convention, Atlanta.

Luper, H. L., and Cross, D. E. 1978. Finger reaction time of stuttering and nonstuttering children and adults. Paper presented at the American Speech and Hearing Association Convention, San Francisco.

McGee, S. R., Hutchinson, J. M., and Deputy, P. N. 1981. The influence of the onset of phonation on the frequency of disfluency among children who stutter. J. Speech Hear. Res. 24:269–272.

Metz, D., Conture, E., and Caruso, A. 1979. Voice onset time, fricative and aspiration durations: A comparison of stutterers and nonstutterers. J. Speech Hear. Res. 22:649–656.

Murphy, M., and Baumgartner, J. M. 1981. Voice initiation and termination time in stuttering and nonstuttering children. J. Fluency Disord. 6:257–264.

Myers, F. L. 1978. Relationship of eight physiological variables and severity of stuttering. J. Fluency Disord. 3:181–191.

Negus, V. W. 1949. The Comparative Anatomy and Physiology of the Larynx. William Heinemann Medical Books, London.

Nelson, L. A. 1982. Evaluation of disfluency, prevention of stuttering, and management of fluency problems in children. Paper presented at the conference sponsored by the Speech Foundation of America, Chicago.

Peiper, A. 1963. Cerebral Function in Infancy and Childhood. Consultants Bureau, New York.

Reich, A., and Till, J. 1981. Reaction time experiments with stuttering and nonstuttering children. Paper presented at the American Speech-Language-Hearing Association Convention, Los Angeles.

Reich, A., Till, J., and Goldsmith, H. 1981. Laryngeal and manual reaction times of stuttering and nonstuttering adults. J. Speech Hear. Res. 24:192–196.

Runyon, C. M., and Bonifant, D. C. 1981. A perceptual comparison: All-voiced versus typical reading passages read by children. J. Fluency Disord. 6:247–256.

Sander, E., 1972. When are speech sounds learned? J. Speech Hear. Disord. 37:55–63.

Shine, R. E. 1980. Direct management of the beginning stutterer. Semin. Speech Lang. Hear. 1:339–350.

Starkweather, C. W. 1982. Stuttering and Laryngeal Behavior: A Review. American Speech-Language-Hearing Association, Monograph no. 21.

Starkweather, C. W., Hirschman, P., and Tannenbaum, R. S. 1976. Latency of vocalization: Stutterers versus nonstutterers. J. Speech Hear. Res. 19:481–492.

Starkweather, C. W., and Myers, M. 1979. The duration of subsegments within the intervocalic intervals of stutterers and nonstutterers. J. Fluency Disord. 4:405–214.

Steer, M. D. 1937. Symptomatologies of young stutterers. J. Speech Disord. 2:3–13.

Stromsta, C. 1965. A spectrographic study of dysfluencies labeled as stuttering by parents. Paper presented at the 13th Congress of the International Society of Logopedics and Phoniatrics. De Therapia Vocis et Loquelae, 1.

Subtelny, J. D. 1957. A cephalometric study of the growth of the soft palate. Plastic Reconstruc. Surg. 16:49–62.

Taylor, I. K. 1966. The properties of stuttered words. J. Verb. Learn. Verb. Behav. 5:112–118.

Wall, M. J., and Pfeuffer, S. 1978. A distinctive feature analysis of stuttered phonemes. Paper presented at the American Speech and Hearing Association Convention, San Francisco.

Wall, M. J., Starkweather, C. W., and Cairns, H. S. 1981. Syntactic influences on stuttering in young child stutterers. J. Fluency Disord. 6:283–298.

Wall, M. J., Starkweather, C. W., and Harris, K. S. 1981. The influence of voicing adjustments on the location of stuttering in the spontaneous speech of young child stutterers. J. Fluency Disord. 6:299–310.

Watson, B. C., and Alfonso, P. J. 1982. A comparison of LRT and VOT values between stutterers and nonstutterers. J. Fluency Disord. 7:219–241.

Watson, B. C., and Alfonso, P. J. 1983. Foreperiod and stuttering severity effects on acoustic laryngeal reaction time. J. Fluency Disord. 8:183–205.

Williams, D. E., Silverman, F. H., and Kools, J. A. 1969. Dysfluency behavior of elementary school stutterers and nonstutterers: Loci of instances of dysfluency. J. Speech Hear. Res. 12:308–318.

Zebrowski, P. M., Conture, E. G., and Cudahy, E. A. 1983. Acoustic analysis of young stutterers' fluency: Preliminary observation. Paper presented at the American Speech-Language-Hearing Convention, Cincinnati.

Zimmermann, G. 1980. Articulatory dynamics of fluent utterances of stutterers and nonstutterers. J. Speech Hear. Res. 23:95–107.

6
Assessment of Childhood Stuttering

ISSUES TO CONSIDER

Several significant issues having theoretical and clinical implications for the management of childhood stuttering need to be considered. By definition, "issues" comprise those indeterminate questions in a field that carry great import but which remain equivocal. Indeterminacy does not imply stagnation. Indeed, researchers' attempts to resolve an issue have often generated and advanced a field, even if the issue itself was not definitively resolved.

Normal Nonfluencies versus Stuttering: A Continuum or a Dichotomy?

The issue of the relation between normal nonfluency and stuttering is manifested on at least two levels—on the terminological level and on a more substantive, theoretical level. Various terms have been used to discuss the components of fluency behavior as they occur in children and in adults. Various terms have also been used to describe "normal" disruptions versus pathological breakdowns in the flow of speech, whether they occur in children or in adults. It is widely acknowledged that normal speech, particularly in children but even in adults, is characterized by a modicum of fluency disruptions. Such disruptions consist of pauses or hesitations, prolongations, false starts, repetitions of various lengths, and parenthetical remarks. A great deal of attention has been paid in the literature to the development of stuttering in children, but a paucity of data exists regarding the development of fluency in normal children. A cogent summary of this literature on the development of normal fluency is, however, provided by Starkweather (1980b).

"Fluency" is used in this book as a generic term to refer to the overall domain of rate behavior in speech and language, recognizing that rate in both normal and pathological speech is characterized by fluency disruptions of varying degrees and types. "Nonfluency" and "disfluency" (or "dysfluency," with the prefix "dys-" carrying the dictionary definition of "pathological" or "ill") are used with greater diversity. We use "nonfluencies" to refer to breaks in the flow of speech that are considered to be within normal limits, and "disfluencies" to refer to those judged to be abnormal.

Various sets of quantitative and qualitative parameters have been proposed for differentiating normal nonfluency from stuttering (e.g., Adams, 1977; Curlee, 1980), and for diagnosing cluttering (Myers, 1982) and other rate disturbances of neurogenic origins (Rosenbek, 1980). An interesting counterpart question can be asked: Given a confirmed stutterer, which instances of fluency disruptions, if any, should or could be called normal? For example, syntactic revisions concomitant with thought revisions during the normal course of conversation are not stuttering even if such fluency disruptions are uttered by a confirmed stutterer. That is, the stutterer as the person must be distinguished from that person's fluency behaviors called stuttering. Fluency disruptions emanating from deliberate syntactic revisions comprise an obvious illustration of the question posed above.

The state of the art is not advanced enough to provide a set of absolute, objective measures for differential diagnosis, although some progress has been made, as discussed in the next section. Until and if a comprehensive set of measures can be drawn up, we will continue to face the issue of whether normal nonfluencies and stuttering lie on a continuum or are dichotomous entities.

Foremost among those who feel that the two domains lie on a continuum is Bloodstein, who has carried this theme through successive decades of thinking and writing (1961, 1970, 1975, 1981). According to Bloodstein, continuity exists between the mild tensions and fragmentations characteristic of the normal speech of youngsters due to "commonplace communicative pressures and difficulties" (1981, p. 300) and the intensification of these fluency disruptions called moments of stuttering. If one were to accept the continuity hypothesis, the task of differential diagnosis would become increasingly difficult as one drew closer to the middle of the continuum, bounded by "normal nonfluency" on one end and "stuttering" marking the opposite end (Myers and Wall, 1981).

Bloodstein (1981, p. 300) credits Wendell Johnson as being one of the first to consider the dichotomous view, although some of Johnson's original research based on parent interviews found overlappings of characteristics shared by stutterers and nonstutterers (Johnson and Associates, 1959). For example, prolongations and part-word repetitions were also prevalent in the speech of some of the nonstutterers, along with some indication of tension and effort associated with their fluency disruptions.

Although the issue of the relation between normal nonfluency and stuttering has not been resolved, it continues to generate much fruitful discussion and research. Its implications are significant, particularly for the differential diagnosis of normal and pathological fluency behavior in children.

Normal Nonfluencies versus Stuttering: Quantitative or Qualitative Differences?

Related to the issue of viewing early childhood stuttering as continuous with or dichotomous from normal childhood nonfluencies is the issue of whether the two domains of behavior are quantitatively or qualitatively different (Myers and Wall, 1981). The quantitative viewpoint reduces the role of intrinsic, qualitative differences and holds that stuttering merely comprises more, in degree as well as severity, of the same types of symptomatology that make up normal childhood nonfluencies. As one moves closer toward the middle of this continuum (with normal nonfluency and stuttering marking the respective poles), the task of differential diagnosis becomes increasingly difficult. Viewing the two clusters of behavior as qualitatively different from each other would lead the clinician to seek features or patterns that distinguish stuttering from normal childhood nonfluencies. In particular, traits such as laryngeal and oral tension (Starkweather, 1982), inappropriate articulatory gestures (Van Riper, 1971), and differences in voice initiation and voice termination times as well as airflow (Adams and Hayden, 1976; Stromsta, 1965) have been offered as distinctive characteristics of stuttering, particularly for the older child stutterer or the adult. Implicit in the qualitative viewpoint is the possibility of two or more inherently distinct subgroups within the stuttering population, with varying symptomatologies and perhaps with different etiologies.

From another perspective, quantitative (rather than qualitative) parameters can be used to differentiate stuttering from nonstuttering behaviors, although both parameters are necessary. A number of quantitative indices, such as stuttered words or syllables per minute, rate of speech, and duration of the longest block, are discussed in the literature. These are bits of behaviors, either for a particular instance of disfluency or across moments of disfluencies, which can be easily, discretely, and segmentally identified and measured.

One must not lose sight, however, of the gestalt in which discrete moments of disfluencies are embedded. The gestalt, containing aspects of the suprasegmentals and other characteristics that are less discrete, provides an important backdrop for judgment of the individual moments of stuttering. These contextual cues include the child's overall "rate, pitch, loudness, inflectional patterns, articulation, facial expression, and postural adjustments . . . [so that] there are stutterers for whom its features are not always confined in an easily identifiable manner to discrete 'moments' " (Bloodstein, 1981, p. 1).

Complicating matters is the perennial awareness of the interaction effect between a child's fluency behavior and the perceiver of that behavior. Even though the human ear is often considered to be the most valid judge of speech and language behaviors, the vagaries of human perception nonetheless influence the validity and reliability of clinical observations. Because human communication in the end is a psychophysical phenomenon, it cannot be measured as exhaustively and precisely as a physical scientist can measure the number of decibels in a sound wave. Thus, taking a gestalt approach to the assessment of childhood stuttering is a judgmental process. As such, it is subject to the vicissitudes of clinician experience and attitudes, the context of the child's communication, inter- and intra-clinician agreement, as well as, of course, the child's communication behavior. The severity as well as type and frequency of the child's stuttering will influence the clinician's judgment. Bloodstein (1981) has defined stuttering in part as ". . . whatever is perceived as stuttering by a reliable observer who has relatively good agreement with others" (p. 9).

All things being equal, a child's disfluencies are more likely to be judged as stuttering: 1) the more severe or effortful the block; 2) the more fragmentary the unit on which the block occurs (Wingate's elemental units of stuttering consisting of sound or syllable repetitions, and sound prolongations); and 3) the greater the frequency of occurrence of fluency disruptions, either during a particular block or across moments of stuttering. For example, if 15% of the words of a speech sample were repeated, even single-unit repetitions tend to be judged as stuttering (Hegde and Hartman, 1979), although single-unit repetitions (e.g., [sə-sʌn]) are normally less likely to be considered as stuttering compared to double-unit repetitions as in [sə-sə-sʌn].

The Heterogeneity of Stuttering and Individual Differences

Until recently, research in the field of communication disorders has been at least indirectly influenced by the popularity of inferential statistics. Focus on group means, as would occur when using inferential statistics, can overshadow the clinical significance of heterogeneity and individual differences as individual raw scores are collapsed to find group means. In inferential statistics, if the number of subjects in the sample is large enough, one can more safely assume that the group mean derived from the group of subjects is representative of the entire population from which this sample was drawn.

Although large n's (n = number of subjects in the sample) often provide power of prediction, some weaknesses inherent in collapsing across subjects might also exist. First, the statistical mean may mask out clinically significant differences across subjects and the existence of subgroups in a population. There are likely to be multiple subgroups of stutterers, reflecting intrinsic differences of etiology and/or symptomatology. A second weakness is that the statistical mean may not be helpful in understanding the fluency problems of a particular child. Owing much to the recent kinds of research, particularly in the field of child language (i.e., in-depth longitudinal studies of a small group of subjects), we have been made more aware of the existence and importance of individual differences and ranges of normality across different children.

Heterogeneity in children's disfluency behavior can be manifested in different ways. Starkweather (1980a), for example, suggested that the various types of stuttering behavior may be due to different conditioning histories. Bloodstein (1981) echoes this viewpoint: "In the final analysis the loci of stutterings seem to have their main source in each stutterer's individual history of learning experiences" (p. 237). McLelland and Cooper (1978) posited that stuttering may represent a more complex phenomenon for males than for females. For example, boys may manifest more severe symptoms even during the early stages of the onset and development of stuttering compared to girls. Myers' (1978) subjects showed great individual differences in eight physiological variables that correlated with the severity of stuttering.

Language-Speech Acquisition and Stuttering: The Delay in Some Stutterers

A fair proportion of children who stutter also exhibit some delay in speech and language development (e.g., Kline and Starkweather, 1979; Westby, 1979). The idea of a relation between language and fluency behaviors in children is gaining momentum, although thinking along these lines is not new. As early as the late 1930's, for example, Davis (1939) found that the word and phrase repetitions of normal preschoolers decreased with age and, presumably, with increased speech and language maturation. In her 1940 study, Davis found negative correlation between the frequency of syllable, word and phrase repetitions and language development (as measured by mean length of response) in nonstutterers.

In spite of this early observation of or at least interest in a possible relation between fluency and language development, the field of communication disorders really had to wait until the discipline of psycholinguistics came into existence in the 1950's and blossomed since the 1960's. The sheer measurement of language development, such as defining and measuring language and then capturing this language in a valid and reliable way, was no easy task. As linguistics and psycholinguistics evolved, one saw a mirroring of developments in our own field. Muma (1971) applied the transformational model of syntax to study the relation between fluency and language behavior in preschoolers. Wall (1980) used phrase structure analysis to compare the syntactic development of a small group of young stutterers and nonstutterers. The current trend of broadening our scope from a piecemeal approach (i.e., looking at stuttering segmentally as if it were largely independent of other aspects of development) to a comprehensive view (i.e., looking at the child from a gestalt communication perspective) has helped to highlight the possible interplay among the various aspects of communication development.

Differential Diagnosis of Normal Nonfluency versus Stuttering

Of critical importance to the differential diagnosis of normal from pathological disfluency is the continuity hypothesis. Even though this issue has
not been resolved, certain fluency behaviors seem to carry more weight in
the direction of what would be considered the pathological than what
would be considered the normal end of the continuum.

An analogy can be drawn between differential diagnosis and probability curves in inferential statistics in that we can talk about levels of
confidence of our clinical judgment. Certain disfluencies have greater
powers of prediction than others for making a prognostic statement about a
disfluent child. To carry this analogy further, portions of the probability
curves for normal nonfluency and for pathological disfluency overlap,
such that behaviors under the normal nonfluency curve can also be exhibited by children diagnosed as stutterers. It seems less likely that behaviors
under the stuttering curve would be shared by normal youngsters. However, even this issue is not clear. McDearmon, for example, in his reexamination of Johnson's data on young stutterers and nonstutterers, found
that of 150 normally fluent children, parents reported that 89.5% exhibited
normal nonfluency, 9.1% exhibited "primary stuttering," and 1.3% exhibited "secondary stuttering." Parents of 150 young stutterers, however, reported that at the onset of stuttering, 30.5% exhibited normal nonfluencies,
65.4% exhibited "primary stuttering," and 4.1% exhibited "secondary stuttering" (McDearmon, 1968, p. 635).

As these various behavioral traits are examined, however, one must be
mindful of the influence of the perceptual set or bias that the listener brings
to the task of differential diagnosis. Curran and Hood (1977), for example,
found that judgments of stuttering severity are related to the number of
repeated units per instance of speech repetition. Sound or syllable repetitions and sound prolongations are more likely to be judged as stuttering
behavior, whereas revisions and interjections are more likely to be considered as normal fluency disruptions (Schiavetti, 1975; Williams and Kent,
1958).

Various classification systems exist for categorizing fluency disruptions in the flow of speech. Johnson (1961) considered the following types:
interjections, part-word repetitions including sound and syllable repetitions, phrase repetitions, revisions (as in "He is——he was"), incomplete
phrases (as in "He was——and then he went"), broken words (as in "He
w—[pause]—as going"), and prolonged sounds. Hood (1978) groups the
various disfluencies into categories such as audible-vocalized (as in part-
word repetitions), audible-nonvocalized (as with sound prolongations),
inaudible-nonvocalized (as with "hard contacts"), and avoidance-escape
(as with "silent pauses"). Hood also categorizes emotions and "behavioral
intentions" related to the moment of stuttering.

The following list of qualitative indices deals with the *manner* (rather than the "quantity") of fluency disruptions that we feel may be prognostic of pathology. These include part-word repetitions and prolongations (Wingate's unitary or elemental stuttering), disrhythmic phonation related to laryngeal tension, tense pauses (i.e., pauses not appropriate to the sense or thought unit of the message), aberrant coarticulatory postures, perception of the schwa during part-word repetitions, frequent difficulty in initiating or sustaining voicing or airflow for speech (Adams, 1980), secondaries, and circumlocutions. By contrast, the behaviors of phrase repetitions, revisions, and interjections are more likely to be associated with normal nonfluencies unless such behaviors occur frequently. Word repetition is considered by some but not all to be a symptom of early stuttering. Van Riper (1982) uses it as one index of stuttering when the word is repeated three or more times.

Regardless of which system of classification one examines, cardinal potency seems to be associated with greater tension, greater fragmentation, greater self-awareness, and greater negative feelings associated with communication. Such traits assist in differentiating the normal from the abnormal.

Van Riper (1982) speaks of negative feelings as the covert features of stuttering and includes anxiety, fear, frustration, hostility, and guilt. These negative feelings are not, of course, necessarily concomitant with the onset of stuttering during early childhood. Nonetheless, the idea that a child consciously or subconsciously associates some set of negative feelings about the pressures of communication is highly germane to the anticipatory struggle theories of the onset of stuttering in childhood. Bluemel (1932), for instance, hypothesized that stuttering results from the child's reactions to his own relatively innocuous fluency disruptions. Bloodstein's theory of communicative failure states that "what is first identified as stuttering usually begins as a response of tension and fragmentation in speech, not sharply different from certain types of normal disfluency, and is brought about largely by the provocation of continued or severe communicative failure in the presence of communicative pressure" (Bloodstein, 1981, p. 56). Therefore, the affective components, such as fear and anxiety, associated with the psychosocial dynamics of communication also must be considered in the process of differential diagnosis.

Various authors have offered quantitative indices to differentiate normal nonfluencies and stuttering. "Quantitative" is used in this section to refer to a numerical index or number of tokens for a particular type of stuttering. Table 1 is a summary of some of the quantitative indices offered in the literature.

The foregoing qualitative and quantitative parameters represent preliminary attempts toward the differential diagnosis of normality from pathology. An area deserving greater attention is differential diagnosis across

Table 1.   Some quantitative indices to differentiate normal from pathological fluency disruptions (selected from authors' list of criteria)

Quantitative indices	Source
10 + disfluencies per 100 words	Adams (1977)
3 + units repetition per part-word repetition	Adams (1980)
1 + sec prolongation on 2% or more of words	Curlee (1980)
1 + sec prolongation per 100 words	Van Riper (1982)
2 + syllable repetitions per word	Van Riper (1982)

various fluency disorders, such as stuttering contrasted with cluttering (Emerick and Hatten, 1979; Myers, 1982). Interestingly, Weiss (1964) aligned cluttering closely with the early stages of stuttering and, indeed, viewed cluttering along the same continuum of fluency disorders as stuttering.

GUIDELINES FOR ASSESSING THE YOUNG STUTTERER: THE GESTALT APPROACH TO ASSESSMENT

In our clinical work we adopt a gestalt approach, examining aspects of the entire communication process pertinent to stuttering. This gestalt approach is accomplished by: 1) proposing a model to organize the assessment process into the psychosocial, physiological, and psycholinguistic factors; 2) viewing communication as a psychosocial phenomenon, to ensure cognizance of the possible interation between the child's disfluencies, his environment, and his subsequent communication behaviors; and 3) assessing both the quantitative and qualitative characteristics of the child's stuttering symptoms.

A Three-Factor Model:
Psychosocial, Physiological, and Psycholinguistic Factors

Our discussion of a set of diagnostic principles for each of the three factors includes a set of specific diagnostic questions to ask during the evaluation. The model set forth earlier now serves as a framework for sorting out the multiplicity of variables to be considered in assessing a child with disfluencies. The set of principles and diagnostic questions posed in this section should be considered *in conjunction* with the matrix of fluency and language behaviors in Table 2 (p. 144) when evaluating the young disfluent child.

Although some of the variables fit neatly and rather exclusively into a particular factor (e.g., genetic predisposition is a physiological factor), other variables (e.g., communicative stress) straddle two or all three factors. That is, the variable of communicative stress, central to the anticipatory struggle hypothesis (Bloodstein, 1981), can conceivably have simultaneous influence on the psychosocial, physiological, and even the psycholinguistic factors. For example, anticipating a difficult communication situation, as when speaking with an intimidating authority figure (psychosocial factor), a young stutterer's coarticulatory skills for speech become less fluent (physiological factor) and simultaneously his linguistic output may be aborted, reduced, or disrupted (psycholinguistic factor).

The Psychosocial Factor   The focal points of the psychosocial factor (Figure 1, Chapter 1) consist of important individuals, both adults and peers, in the child's daily environment. Perhaps the most central figures are the child's parents. Several major hypotheses that have had a profound impact on our field have highlighted the role of parents in the etiology of stuttering. In particular, Johnson's diagnosogenic theory states that stuttering emanates from the parents' ill perception and subsequent judgment of the child's normal nonfluencies as stuttering. This theory has directly or indirectly influenced clinicians' postures regarding the management of early childhood disfluencies for the past several decades. Only in relatively recent times have clinicians begun to adopt a more direct therapy approach for youngsters (e.g., Ryan, 1974; Shine, 1980; Stocker, 1980).

A more inclusive theory pertinent to the psychosocial factor is the interaction hypothesis offered by Johnson (Johnson and Associates, 1959). This hypothesis highlights the significance of both the interpersonal and the intrapersonal variables to be considered under the psychosocial factor.

Congruent with the trend toward more direct attention to the young stutterer are research findings that even preschoolers can have intuitions about their own or other children's disfluencies. Langer (1969) found that first through fourth graders can differentiate at least on a general level fluent from highly disfluent speech. Although parents sometimes say that "Children can be cruel," it is also likely that some of the reactions of youngsters toward stuttering may initially reflect curiosity toward the unknown or the different.

Just as important as the interpersonal dynamics discussed above are the intrapersonal dynamics of stuttering. That is, how does the child view himself and his speech? Awareness of speech difficulties serves as a major demarcation between Phases 1 and 2 of Bloodstein's schema and between the primary and secondary stages of Bluemel's schema for the development of stuttering. When signs of awareness are evident, childlike but fitting terms such as "hard speech" or "bumpy speech" or "getting stuck" might be used by the child or the clinician to describe this awareness.

Diagnostic questions related to the psychosocial factor:

1. Does the child "know" he sometimes has fluency disruptions?

The quotation marks around "know" indicate that different children manifest such awareness in different ways, ranging from the most nebulous and fleeting intuitions to explicit verbalization about the disfluencies. From the Piagetian literature, clinicians should also be sensitive to children's varying capacities for knowledge and for differentiating self from the environment. Awareness, when present in a child, may manifest itself in speech or nonspeech behaviors, such as avoiding social interactions containing a high degree of communicative stress.

2. If the child seems to know that he sometimes has fluency disruptions, in what ways, to what extent, and when does he react to these disfluencies?

Put in another way, this diagnostic question probes *how, to what extent*, and *in what types of pragmatic situations* does the child react? The degree of reactions should be gauged both at the speech level and at the affective level. Ultimately, especially for the more severe child stutterer, such probes are aimed toward estimating the amount of control the child feels as he experiences momentary communicative breakdowns.

3. How does the child's fluency behavior affect his parents?

It is critical during the diagnostic interview to get a thorough assessment of the parents' perception of stuttering and their specific behavioral descriptions of the child's disfluencies. We have found that the term "stuttering" tends more to be overused than underused by parents. It is best to have the parents simulate examples of their child's disfluencies during the parent interview, followed by joint observations of their child's communication behavior behind a one-way mirror, as the child interacts with another clinician and/or another child in the therapy room.

During this observation period, the descriptors first provided by the parents can then be substantiated and/or elaborated. We have found the coupling of these two parts of the diagnostic session to be a very useful and powerful medium for parent counseling.

4. How do the parents' communication behaviors influence the child?

In addition to the parents' reaction to the child's speech and language, the clinician should observe the reactions and the interactions of the child as a function of the parents' communication behaviors. Whereas investigators such as Snow (1972) have examined child-adult interactions in the broader context of child language development and disorders, L. J. Johnson (1980), Starkweather (1983, personal communication), and Prins (1983) have specifically focused on the topic of parental communication style and the child stutterer. Aspects of parents' communication include speech rate, relative degree of tension accompanying speech production (even though fluent), turn-taking styles, amount and types of questions asked, degree of emotional content of utterances, and linguistic complexity of the adults' conversational input.

5. Finally, how is the child's overall adjustment to himself, to his speech, and to the reactions of others?

Human beings, young and old, seek equilibrium. Depending on the degree of awareness, successive moments of blocks can momentarily tip the child off balance. In their own individual ways, whether it is during the speech act or through other behaviors and feelings related to communication, stutterers attempt to regain equilibrium. It is important to observe how the child attempts to do this. It is also critical to realize that different youngsters have different thresholds of tolerance for factors that disrupt this equilibrium. Some children are highly sensitive, whereas others are mildly or negligibly sensitive. In keeping with the gestalt approach, the diagnostician must therefore take stock of the various inter- and intrapersonal forces that impinge on the child during moments of disfluency or even during periods of fluency.

The Physiological Factor   Chapter 5 discussed in detail the physiological aspects of childhood stuttering. Now we focus on assessment of the physiological aspects of the speech production system, following the traditional headings of respiration, phonation, and coarticulation and the aerodynamics of the vocal tract. Although resonance is important for speech production, its role in fluency is minimal. For each of the speech production processes, a set of principles is followed by a set of specific diagnostic questions to be used in assessing the speech of a disfluent child.

Respiration   The literature has not found that the respiratory mechanism itself is faulty in stutterers. Aberrant breathing is likely to reflect a secondary or tertiary level effect resulting from poor coordination between control of the upcoming airstream and one or more of the following: laryngeal control, coarticulatory and aerodynamic modulations, or the length and complexity of the language unit being encoded. Such harmony needs to be well tuned, well timed, well coordinated, and well sequenced.

Some specific diagnostic questions include the following:

1.   Is there evidence of shallow breathing?

2. Are the respiratory cycles irregular, jerky, or excessively aperiodic?

3. Is the inspiratory or the expiratory phase periodically aborted?

4. Is there a lack of coordination between the child's breathing pattern and the phonatory, coarticulatory/aerodynamic, or linguistic subcomponents of his communicative attempts?

Phonation   The research literature (see St. Louis, 1979, for a summary of the recent research) has pointed to the importance of an efficient and effective phonatory mechanism, contributing to the following functions: smooth reciprocity of laryngeal abduction and adduction, optimal range of overall laryngeal tension, and synergy between phonation and the other aspects of speech production. A great deal of interest in the detailed study of voicing characteristics (VOT, VIT, VTT) of children and adults notwithstanding (e.g., Cullinan and Springer, 1980; Conture, 1982, personal communication regarding ongoing research), the clinician does not have ready access to the sophisticated instrumentation necessary to assess a young disfluent child's laryngeal behavior. Nevertheless, perceptual traits such as those listed below can be examined:

1. Is the child's phonatory quality aberrant (e.g., occasional harshness, vocal fry, unusually high pitch, or loud vocal tone)?

2. Does the child exhibit silent blocks (during production of a lexical item) or tense pauses (between lexical items)?

3. Does the child show disrhythmic phonation during prolongation of sounds?

4. Does the child show hard glottal attacks?

5. Is there evidence of rapidly fluctuating pitch levels during syllable repetitions?

Coarticulatory and Aerodynamic Factors   McDonald (1964) defines coarticulation as a series of highly coordinated, overlapping movements (due to the influence of phonetic contexts) that provides changing degrees of obstruction in the way of the outgoing airstream and at the same time changes the size, shape, and coupling of the resonating cavities.

The essence of coarticulation then is the temporal overlapping of articulatory movements for different sounds (Borden and Harris, 1980). Looking at the vocal tract as a series of valves, indeed one can appreciate the intricacies requisite for the modulation of the airflow and air pressure needed for ongoing speech.

Stuttering is often thought of as involving an excess of muscular tension so that the valving mechanism, as when the lips approximate to make the plosive /p/, shows hyperfunction and/or incoordination resulting in the inability to release air after bilabial closure. A stuttering child may or may not have an articulatory problem in addition to the coarticulatory and aerodynamic problems associated with his fluency difficulties. Van Riper's definition of stuttering as difficulty with the coarticulatory transitions between sounds sensitizes us to the importance of smooth and appropriate transitions between sounds. He cites the prevalence of the schwa during syllable repetitions as symptomatic of difficulties with making the coarticulatory transitions, as in [bə-, bə-, beɪbi]. It is as if the stutterer perseverates on the schwa until he has landed on the correct transition.

Some diagnostic questions to consider during assessment include the following:

1. Does the child appear to have difficulty in making transitions between sounds (e.g., presence of schwa)?
2. Is there improper or excessive valving somewhere along the vocal tract, looking at the speech production system as a neuromuscular aerodynamic system?
3. Is there excessive supraglottal air pressure?
4. Is there improper control or modulation of air pressure and airflow during speech?

Summary Remarks   Again reinforcing the notion of a gestalt approach to assessing the young stutterer, it is apparent from the foregoing discussion that the various processes of the speech production mechanism should be viewed from a systems approach. Subcomponents of the system are coordinated with and influence each other such that a breakdown in one part of the system could effect another part of the system. The synergism of respiration with phonation and coarticulation is especially pertinent in reference to time because speech is an ongoing and relatively fleeting process. This point leads us to Van Riper's central concept of stuttering as a disorder of the temporal aspects of speech, emphasizing that speech is patterned in time.

Stuttering results when the sequencing of syllables is disrupted in time. The synchrony of movements is needed, for example, to govern the timing of speech sounds relative to pauses in speech, and of the suprasegmentals as they are superimposed on syllables. In reviewing the literature on the linguistic and motor aspects of stuttering, St. Louis (1979) states that one persepective of stuttering is in terms of "defects in the precise timing of respiration and phonation which, in turn, generate the complex supraglottal articulatory symptoms" (p. 152).

Two final, precautionary notes are in order. First, because relatively more research has been done on adult stutterers than on children, it is tempting to apply such findings directly to the fluency problems of children. Direct transfer of adult findings to children may not be warranted, however. Second, although findings on adults may provide food for thought about the child stutterer, it remains to be seen whether the behavioral symptoms discussed in this section for the assessment of childhood stuttering can be interpreted as the cause of stuttering or as the surface symptomatology of the disorder.

The Psycholinguistic Factor   There is much current interest in the relation between fluency and language development, although superficial observations of the presence of such a relationship were noted decades ago by Davis (1939, 1940). Of course, a great deal has transpired in the field of child language since the 1940's. In fact psycholinguistics itself did not exist until the mid-1950's. Chapter 4 provides a brief historical perspective of the field of developmental psycholinguistics, and overviews the current methodological approaches to the study of child language.

The past decade has witnessed in the field of developmental psycholinguistics some exciting work, both on the theoretical/research as well as on the clinical fronts. Continued fine-tuning of the field of developmental psycholinguistics is necessary to elaborate upon the nature of the relation between language and fluency. The ultimate direction of this fine-tuning remains to be seen. Chapter 4 offers some insight into the possible relations between language and fluency.

Language has traditionally been thought of in terms of syntax, semantics, and pragmatics. With Chapter 4 as background reading, the following diagnostic questions should be considered during the assessment of a disfluent child.

Syntax

1. Does the child have a syntax delay or deficit in addition to his fluency problem?

2. Does the child experience fluency breakdowns especially with the syntactically more complex utterances he is attempting to formulate?

3. If so, as when attempting to encode several ideas using a complex or complex-compound sentence, where does the child experience such breakdowns?

The question of "where" refers to the loci of disfluency, and all things being equal, the loci of early childhood stuttering has been shown to be at the beginnings of clauses and phrases (Bloodstein, 1974). The loci for later childhood and adult stuttering, on the other hand, seem to be more word-bound (Williams, Silverman, and Kools, 1969).

4. What types of speech behavior does the child manifest during these moments of fluency breakdown?

In contrast to question 3, dealing with the location of breakdown, this question refers to the manner of breakdown. All things being equal, the more fragmentary and tense the moment of disfluency, the more severe it tends to be regarded. Wingate (1976) refers to the distinguishing features of sound/syllable repetitions and prolongations as "unitary" or "elemental," and points to these types of speech behavior as the core or the essence of stuttering.

Semantics

1. Is there a relation between the child's disfluency and the sophistication of the cognitive notions underlying the child's semantic intent?

Various systems of analyzing a child's semantic intent in an utterance are available (e.g., Bloom and Lahey, 1978; MacDonald and Nickols, 1974). Whichever system is chosen, the clinician can superimpose a schema for the simultaneous analysis of the child's fluency pattern. A child who is predominantly at Phase 4 of Bloom and Lahey's form/content categories, for example, may show a particular increase in disfluencies as he attempts to encode semantic content categories in Phase 5. Such information would have diagnostic as well as therapeutic implications, as when contrasted with another child whose disfluency patterns were not bound by a semantic ceiling but permeated his earlier as well as later semantic categories.

Although we have observed patterns such as those described above in our own clinical experience, this entire area would benefit from closer scrutiny in research.

2. Is there a pattern of fluency breakdown corresponding to the degree of information load carried by individual lexical items?

"Information load," a term favored by theorists dealing with cybernetics and communication theory, is based on forward-guessing techniques whereby subjects are asked to predict the next occurring word. The greater the probability that a word will be guessed, the less information that word presumably carries. A high degree of probability exists for predicting the word "eggs" (hence the less information carried) in "bacon and _____," than predicting the word in "I am going to _____." Content words have generally been considered to carry higher information load than the "little" function words of the English language such as *a, the, and,* and indeed the general finding seems to be that at least older children stutter more on content than on function words because the former carry more meaning (Williams, Silverman, and Kools, 1969). (See Bloodstein and Gantwerk,

1967, however, for a discussion of the complex interaction between grammatical class of words and the position effect of words for the disfluencies of early childhood stuttering.)

3. Is there a pattern of fluency breakdown as a function of the degree of propositionality of an utterance?

This question overlaps a great deal with question 2 about information load, because it is difficult to tease apart the variables of meaningfulness, information load, and the degree of communicative responsibility taken on by a speaker in an utterance. Because the perception of communicative stress by children is central to his thinking about the etiology and development of stuttering, Bloodstein (1981) discusses communicative responsibility (which includes the meaningfulness or propositionality of speech) as being influenced by the form and content of the stutterer's message, the listener, and the psychosocial context of the message. All things being equal, one would predict less disfluencies accompanying reduced propositionality or reduced psychosocial load of the discourse interaction. This leads us to the next area of language for clinical investigation, pragmatics.

Pragmatics   Pragmatics deals with the use of language in varying psychosocial contexts. It is an aspect of communication that covers a broad spectrum of skills, including those needed for the appropriate gauging of presuppositions, for the use of polite forms, and for making requests. Of the several areas of language development under discussion, pragmatics is probably the most vulnerable to the vicissitudes and flux of interpersonal and intrapersonal dynamics.

1. What is the psychosocial context of the discourse in which the child is exhibiting his fluency behavior?

The psychosocial context incorporates variables related to the child, the listener, and the speaking situation; and each of these factors interfaces with the others. Silverman (1971), for example, found that her 4-year-old normals were more nonfluent in a structured interview situation than in less structured situations such as at home or at their preschool. Particularly in view of the current trend in communication assessment of looking at the child's speech and language in low structured naturalistic settings, the clinician must be cognizant of the influence that the assessment situation can exert over the child's fluency behavior.

2. What are the types and frequencies of pragmatic functions exhibited in the child's speech sample, and how do such functions affect the child's stuttering?

Some pragmatic functions such as the "personal" function may be more innocuous than others, such as the "regulatory" and "instrumental" functions that are motivated by the child's attempt to control someone else's behavior.

3. Is there any interaction effect between pragmatic variables and the length and complexity of the child's syntax?

Clinicians should be mindful that utterances of the same length and syntactic complexity may produce different fluency profiles as a function of different pragmatic intents and discourse settings.

In summary, this section of the chapter has sought to heighten clinician's awareness of the potential impact of a child's syntactic, semantic, and pragmatic skills on his fluency behavior. The clinician might also consider the possibility of phonological influences on fluency, as discussed in Chapter 4.

The Moment of Stuttering:
Its Complexity

As discussed in Chapter 3, various behavioral dimensions can be considered when analyzing specific moments of stuttering. The word "behavioral" is used in a broad sense to include a wide host of symptoms, some of which are more readily observable than others. The existence of symptoms that are not readily observable has serious clinical as well as research implications.

On the diagnostic level, some subtle bits of behavior, particularly in the laryngeal area, may project potent prognostic insights were the clinician able to pick up on these cues. By the same token, perhaps some stutterers have been dismissed from therapy because they sounded "fluent" but who nonetheless harbored minute traits of disfluencies. Adams and Runyan (1981), when referring to the idea of "tenuous stuttering," discussed the possibility that stutterers' so-called fluent speech may also be marked by longer VOT, discontinuities in voicing between words, slight rises in modal fundamental frequency, or discontinuities in voicing between words. Adams and Runyan advocate a three-stage model to characterize a stutterer's speech that includes his stuttering, his "tenuous fluency," and his fluency. On the research level, likewise, failure to pick up these subtle but nonetheless potentially significant aspects of fluency behavior may have led researchers to include occasional instances of "tenuously fluent" speech as "fluent" speech.

Two major dimensions, the visible and the audible, can be used to describe the overt manifestations of a stuttering response. These two dimensions can occur alone or together. For example, a syllable repetition is at once audible and visible. Some authors superimpose on these two dimensions a third dimension, namely, the contrasting of the primary with the secondary or associated symptoms of stuttering. Regardless of which dimensions are used, an additional critical element would be to assess the child's disfluencies in the context of normal developmental patterns of fluency, rate and pause time (Starkweather, 1980b).

In addition to the so-called integral or essential features of stuttering (repetitions, prolongations, and tense pauses), the associated or secondary characteristics of stuttering are also important. The complexity of studying the moment of stuttering is again highlighted by the acknowledgment that these associated symptoms are difficult to confine in a neat, discrete matrix because stutterers vary in their symptomatology and because some of the associated features are not overt. Examples of the latter include certain physiological correlates of stuttering (Myers, 1978) and the stutterers' perception of others and of themselves during moments of stuttering (Bloodstein, 1981).

Overt, perceptible associated symptoms include eye blinks, nares dilation, and head jerks; as with the core characteristics of stuttering, these can be quantitatively as well as qualitatively assessed. The associated symptoms are most often seen in older, severe stutterers. Hood (1978) includes an additional dimension labeled "behavioral intentions" to characterize the moment of stuttering, but rightfully acknowledges the difficulty of detecting, for example, "whether the intention of a short pause was related to linguistic encoding behavior as opposed to avoidance and postponement related to stuttering . . . [or] . . . whether the intention of such behavior represented a short silent pause or a brief, silent fixation of articulation posture" (Hood, 1978, p. 555). Such "behavioral intentions" are very much intermeshed with one's feelings and perceptions toward oneself and toward others.

The complexity of stuttering responses warrants the exercise of caution in their analysis. Once moments of stuttering can be identified, the task remains of somehow drawing patterns of disfluencies across successive moments of stuttering. The second leg of this assessment task is perhaps less complicated than the specification of individual overt and covert stuttering responses. Patterns can be extracted in terms of the rated severity, the frequency, the loci and distribution, and the average and range of durations of blocks. Frequency can be tapped by such means as percentage of words stuttered or percentage of syllables stuttered, stuttered words per minute, and number of units of repetitions per moment of block. For example, [bə- bə- beɪbi] contains two units of repetition on the first syllable. Because the fluency disruptions exhibited by a stutterer can contain elements of both normal nonfluency (e.g., change in thought during an utterance) and those attributable to stuttering, the clinician must specify whether the numerical indices cited above are based on the latter only or on both types of fluency disruption.

Loci patterns refer to the location of disfluency, whether it be in the context of the stuttered word itself or in a larger context such as a phrase, clause, or sentence. The seminal and influential study on adults by Brown (1945) found, based on statistical analyses, four factors influencing the loci of stuttering: word length, word position in a sentence, and the initial sound and grammatical function of the word. Chapter 3 reviews the literature pertinent to loci and distribution patterns of stuttering of early and later childhood stuttering. This body of literature illustrates the distinction between findings on the adult or the older child stutterer and on the early childhood stutterer. In general, early childhood stuttering is characterized by loci at the beginning of syntactic units and on function words such as pronouns and conjunctions (which also happen to prevail frequently at the beginnings of syntactic units). The distribution of disfluency shifts away from the initiation of syntactic units and becomes more word bound for later childhood stutterers, to parallel the kinds of pattern observed in adult stutterers.

Situational Factors in the Assessment of Childhood Stuttering

Lois Bloom's initial and fundamental contribution to the field of child language was to alert clinicians and researchers to the importance of contextual cues for the interpretation of children's utterances. The current trend to provide a low structured and naturalistic environment for language sampling prevails in order to obtain a representative and valid sample of the child's language (e.g., Bloom and Lahey, 1978). However, this approach also imposes a great onus on the clinician to ensure that the context is indeed "representative" and that the "rich interpretation" of the child's utterances is made validly and reliably.

By the same token, assessment of a disfluent child's speech and language also must take into account the variables of representativeness, naturalness, and degrees of linguistic and nonlinguistic structure imposed on the child. These variables in turn are influenced by whether the child's stuttering is assessed during reading or conversation, the child's perception of the listener and the context of discourse, the amount of information load and degree of propositionality of the message, and the degree of linguistic complexity called for in the particular discourse situation. Sensitivity to the psychosocial context of speaking situations starts to be developed at an early age, as exemplified by Shatz and Gelman (1973), who found that 4-year-olds spontaneously adopt different speaking styles when addressing 2-year-olds, their peers, and adults. For example, the subjects were more direct with the younger children than with the other two groups of listeners. These pragmatic sensitivities are bound to have impact on the fluency behaviors of children, regardless of the level of proficiency in the other areas of linguistic development.

Table 2.   Matrix of stuttering behaviors

Name:_____   Clinician:_____
Age:_____   Activities/Discourse Context:_____
Date:_____

I.   **General information**

Size of corpus: No. syllables_____   No. morphemes_____
                 No. words   _____   No. utterances _____

Mean length of utterance in morphemes (if appropriate)   _____

Stuttering
Percentage syllables stuttered $= \dfrac{\text{no. syllables stuttered}}{\text{total no. syllables}} \times 100$ _____

Stuttered syllables per min $= \dfrac{\text{no. syllables stuttered}}{\text{no. minutes}}$ _____

Stuttered words per min $= \dfrac{\text{no. words stuttered}}{\text{no. minutes}}$ _____

   Overall rating of stuttering (7 point rating scale)[a]   ____
   Overall degree of awareness of stuttering (7 point rating scale)[a]   ____
   Overall degree of use of avoidance behaviors (7 point rating
   scale)[a]   ____
   Loci and distribution of stuttering
      Predominantly word bound   ____
      Predominantly clause bound   ____
      Both word and clause bound   ____

II.   **Core behaviors of stuttering**

Percentage sound   _____ Average no. sound repetitions/   ____
   repetitions[b]   word[c]
                                        Range of no. sound repetitions/ ____
                                          word

Percentage syllable   _____ Ave. no. syllable repetitions/   ____
   repetitions[b]   word[c]
                                        Range of syllable repetitions/   ____
                                          word

Percentage word   _____ Ave. no. word repetitions/   ____
   repetitions[b]   word[c]
                                        Range of word repetitions/
                                          word   ____

Percentage phrase   _____ Ave. no. phrase repetitions/   ____
   repetitions[b]   word[c]
                                        Range of phrase repetitions/   ____
                                          word

Percentage sound   _____ Ave. duration of prolongations   ____
   prolongations[b]
                                        Range of duration of   ____
                                          prolongations
Percentage tense pauses or silent blocks (inaudible fixations   _____
   of laryngeal or articulatory posture)[b]

III. Accompanying symptoms of stuttering

Reactions to core behaviors of stuttering[a]

Respiratory disruptions	_____
Vowel glide	_____
Vocal fry	_____
Intensity/pitch disruptions	_____
Phonatory stoppage	_____
Schwa vowel	_____
Facial tension/struggle	_____
Fixed articulatory posture	_____
Body/limb movements	_____

Reactions to fear of stuttering[a]

Postponement (behaviors to defer the onset of a feared word)	_____
Starters (behaviors to help initiation of a feared word)	_____
Avoidance (behaviors to avoid stuttering)	
Gives up speech attempt	_____
Word substitutions, revisions, and circumlocutions	_____
Loss of eye contact	_____
Uses unusual ways of speaking (e.g., chant)	_____
Antiexpectancies/disguise reactions (e.g., assuming another role or manner of speaking)	_____

Based largely on Van Riper's (1982, Chapter Six) description of the overt features of stuttering.

[a]The 7 point rating scale is based on judgment of the relative overall severity and frequency of the stuttering behavior(s) observed. The following descriptors are associated with points on the scale:

0 No stuttering
1 Very mild
2 Mild
3 Mild to moderate
4 Moderate
5 Moderate to severe
6 Severe
7 Very severe

[b]Of the total instances of disfluencies, the percentage that consisted of sound, syllable, word, and phrase repetitions; and the percentage that consisted of sound prolongations and tense pauses or silent blocks. For example:

$$\% \text{ sound repetition} = \frac{\text{no. different instances of sound repetition}}{\text{total no. disfluencies}} \times 100$$

[c]Of the total instances of sound, syllable, word, or phrase repetitions, the average number and range of such repetitions in each category. For example, "be- be- baby" has two repetitions of the first syllable. If the child had the repertoire of syllable repetitions shown below, the average number of syllable repetitions per word is 2.5 and the range of syllable repetitions per word is 1–4.

Total instances of syllable repetitions:

be- be- baby	(2-unit repetition)
Si- Si- Si- Simon	(3-unit repetition)
ma- magic	(1-unit repetition)
so- so- so- so- sofa	(4-unit repetition)

$$\bar{X} = \frac{10 \text{ units}}{4 \text{ words}} = 2.5$$

(Repetitions of monosyllabic words should be put under the category of word repetitions.)

A Matrix for Analyzing Childhood Stuttering

The matrix in Table 2 integrates the various bits of disfluency behaviors into an organized framework. The matrix is to be used in conjunction with the set of diagnostic principles and questions given earlier in the chapter. The behaviors listed in the matrix are not new and indeed represent variations on similar themes offered by other authors (e.g., Emerick and Hatten, 1979; Hood, 1978; Van Riper, 1982; Williams, 1978). For each of the behaviors listed in Table 2, it is important to discern the temporal dynamics of moments of stuttering; that is, the clinician should note the speech and nonspeech behaviors of the child immediately before, during, and immediately after a block. The same set of temporal dynamics should be examined for the speech and nonspeech behaviors of the child's conversational partners. It is very helpful in the clinical management of a child stutterer to have the parents keep a log detailing when and how their child's disfluencies occur and the circumstances around these disfluencies.

CONCLUSION:
SOME PRINCIPLES FOR "PULLING IT TOGETHER"

1. Take a gestalt approach to assessing the child stutterer by: a) considering the psychosocial, physiological, and psycholinguistic factors and the interactions thereof that influence the onset, development, and reduction of stuttering in children; b) assessing the child in the larger context of viewing overall communication skills rather than only evaluating fluency behaviors; and c) assessing both the quantitative and qualitative characteristics of the child's fluent and disfluent speech.

2. Be attuned to the influence of listener and situation variables during the evaluation of childhood stuttering. The clinician and the diagnostic setting are important, intrinsic aspects of the interaction and may directly affect the fluency patterns gathered during the evaluation. Such variables include whether the assessment setting is high- or low-structured, naturalistic or formal, and whether the clinician conveys an unrushed, interested, and supportive approach to the child.

3. Aim for high reliability and precision in quantifying and qualifying the child's fluency behavior.

4. Recognize and optimize the contributions that parents can provide during the evaluation and throughout therapy. We often try to speak to the parents before the diagnostic session, primarily to see whether the child "knows" about his "stuttering." Such information not only gives the clinician a head start but also provides invaluable information for devising the appropriate context for interactions with the child. Given sufficient background information and support, parents can be our best allies in helping to provide continual monitoring of the child's disfluencies, although the kinds of observation made by parents need not be as specific as those made by the clinician.

When the child comes for his initial diagnostic session the clinician will not, of course, have had an opportunity to discuss with the parents the kinds of fluency breakdown the child is experiencing. Nevertheless, the constellation of information, insights, and feelings the parents bring with them during this initial interview hold high diagnostic value, even if parental insights are not initially precise or complete.

The final decisions regarding management of the child's stuttering must be made in consultation with the parent. Furthermore, the ensuing dialogues between clinician and parents should be conducted at both the didactic and the affective levels.

REFERENCES

Adams, M. 1977. A clinical strategy for differentiating the normal nonfluent child and the incipient stutterer. J. Fluency Disord. 2:141–148.

Adams, M. 1980. The young stutterer: Diagnosis, treatment and assessment of progress. Semin. Speech, Lang. Hear. 1:289–298.

Adams, M., and Hayden, P. 1976. The ability of stutterers and nonstutterers to initiate and terminate phonation during the production of an isolated vowel. J. Speech Hear. Res. 19:290–296.

Adams, M., and Runyan, C. 1981. Stuttering and fluency: Exclusive events or points on a continuum. J. Fluency Disord. 6:197–218.

Bloodstein, O. 1961. The development of stuttering. III. Theoretical and clinical implications. J. Speech Hear. Disord. 26:67–82.

Bloodstein, O. 1970. Stuttering and normal nonfluency—A continuity hypothesis. Br. J. Disord. Commun. 5:30–39.

Bloodstein, O. 1974. The rules of early stuttering. J. Speech Hear. Disord. 39:379–394.

Bloodstein, O. 1975. Stuttering as tension and fragmentation. In: J. Eisenson (ed.), Stuttering: A Second Symposium, pp. 1–95. Harper & Row, New York.

Bloodstein, O. 1981. A Handbook on Stuttering. 3rd Ed. National Easter Seal Society, Chicago.

Bloodstein, O., and Gantwerk, B. 1967. Grammatical function in relation to stuttering in young children. J. Speech Hear. Res. 10:786–789.

Bloom, L., and Lahey, M. 1978. Language Development and Language Disorders. John Wiley & Sons, New York.

Bluemel, C. 1932. Primary and secondary stammering. Q. J. Speech. 18:187–200.

Borden, G., and Harris, K. 1980. Speech Science Primer: Physiology, Acoustics, and Perception of Speech. Williams & Wilkins Company, Baltimore.

Brown, S. 1945. The loci of stutterings in the speech sequence. J. Speech Disord. 10:181–192.

Colburn, N. 1979. Disfluency behavior and emerging linguistic structures in preschool children. Unpublished doctoral dissertation, Columbia University, New York.

Cooper, E. 1978. Facilitating parental participation in preparing the therapy component of the stutterer's individualized education program. J. Fluency Disord. 3:221–228.

Cullinan, W., and Springer, M. 1980. Voice initiation times in stuttering and nonstuttering children. J. Speech Hear. Res. 23:344–360.

Curlee, R. 1980. A case selection strategy for young disfluent children. Semin. Speech Lang. Hear. 1:277–287.

Curran, M., and Hood, S. 1977. Listener ratings of severity for specific disfluency types in children. J. Fluency Disord. 2:87–97.

Davis, D. 1939. The relation of repetitions in the speech of young children to certain measures of language maturity and situational factors. Part I. J. Speech Disord. 4:303–318.

Davis, D. 1940. The relation of repetitions in the speech of young children to certain measures of language maturity and situational factors. Parts II and III. J. Speech Disord. 5:235–246.

Emerick, L., and Hatten, J. 1979. Diagnosis and Evaluation in Speech Pathology. 2nd Ed. Prentice-Hall, Englewood Cliffs, N.J.

Hegde, M., and Hartman, D. 1979. Factors affecting judgments of fluency. II. Word repetitions. J. Fluency Disord. 4:13–22.

Hood, S. 1978. The assessment of fluency disorders. In: S. Singh and J. Lynch (eds.), Diagnostic Procedures in Hearing, Language, and Speech, pp. 529–632. University Park Press, Baltimore.

Johnson, L. J. 1980. Facilitating parental involvement in therapy of the disfluent child. Semin. Speech Lang. Hear. 1:4, 301–309.

Johnson, W. 1961. Measurements of oral reading and speaking rate and disfluency of adult male and female stutterers and nonstutterers. J. Speech Hear. Disord. (Monogr. Suppl. 7):1–20.

Johnson, W., and Associates. 1959. The Onset of Stuttering. University of Minnesota Press, Minneapolis.

Kline, M., and Starkweather, C. 1979. Receptive and expressive language performance in young stutterers. Am. Speech Hear. Assoc. 21(abstr.)797.

Langer, R. 1969. A clinical study of the reactions of preschool children to stuttered and non-stuttered speech in another child. Speech Monogr. 36(abstr.):286.

MacDonald, J., and Nickols, M. 1974. Environmental Language Inventory: A semantic-based assessment for training generalized communication. Nisonger Center of Ohio State University, Columbus.

McDearmon, J. 1968. Primary stuttering at the onset of stuttering: A reexamination of data. J. Speech Hear. Res. 11:631–637.

McDonald, E. 1964. Articulation Testing and Treatment: A Sensory-Motor Approach. Stanwyx House, Pittsburgh.

McLelland, J., and Cooper, E. 1978. Fluency-related behaviors and attitudes of 178 young stutterers. J. Fluency Disord. 3:253–263.

Muma, J. 1971. Syntax of preschool fluent and disfluent speech: A transformational analysis. J. Speech Hear. Res. 14:428–441.

Myers, F. 1978. Relationship between eight physiological variables and severity of stuttering. J. Fluency Disord. 3:181–191.

Myers, F. 1982. Acoustic and perceptual characteristics of cluttering. Paper presented at the 22nd Annual Convention of the New York State Speech-Language-Hearing Association, April 25–28, Ellenville, N.Y.

Myers, F., and Wall, M. 1981. Issues to consider in the differential diagnosis of normal childhood nonfluencies and stuttering. J. Fluency Disord. 6:189–195.

Prins, D. 1983. Continuity, fragmentation, and tension: Hypotheses applied to evaluation and intervention with preschool disfluent children. In: D. Prins and R. Ingham (eds.), Treatment of Stuttering in Early Childhood: Methods and Issues, pp. 21–38. College-Hill Press, San Diego.

Rosenbek, J. 1980. Apraxia of speech—Relationship to stuttering. J. Fluency Disord. 5:233–253.

Ryan, B. 1974. Programmed Therapy for Stuttering in Children and Adults. Charles C Thomas Publisher, Springfield, Ill.

Schiavetti, N. 1975. Judgments of stuttering severity as a function of type and locus of disfluency. Fol. Phoniatr. 27:26–37.

Shatz, M., and Gelman, R. 1973. The Development of Communicative Skills: Modifications in the Speech of Young Children as a Function of the Listener. Monograph of Society for Research in Child Development, Vol. 38, no. 152.

Shine, R. 1980. Direct management of the beginning stutterer. Semin. Speech Lang. Hear. 1:339–350.

Silverman, E.-M. 1971. Situational variability of preschoolers' disfluency: A preliminary study. Percept. Motor Skills. 33:1021–1022.

Snow, C. 1972. Mothers' speech to children learning language. Child Devel. 43:549–565.

Starkweather, C. 1980a. A multiprocess behavioral view of stuttering therapy. Semin. Speech Lang. Hear. 1(4):327–338.

Starkweather, C. 1980b. Speech fluency and its development in normal children. In: N. Lass (ed.), Speech and Language: Advances in Basic Research and Practice, pp. 143–200, Vol. 4. Academic Press, New York.

Starkweather, C. 1982. Stuttering and Laryngeal Behavior: A Review. ASHA Monograph no. 21. American Speech-Language-Hearing Association.

St. Louis, K. 1979. Linguistic and motor aspects of stuttering. In: N. Lass (ed.), Speech and Language: Advances in Basic Research and Practice, pp. 89–210. Vol. 1. Academic Press, New York.

Stocker, B. 1980. Stocker Probe Technique: For Diagnosis and Treatment of Stuttering in Young Children. Modern Education Corporation, Tulsa.

Stromsta, C. 1965. A spectrographic study of disfluencies labeled as stuttering by parents. Paper presented at the 13th Congress of the International Society of Logopedics and Phoniatrics. De Therapia Vocis et Loquelae, 1.

Van Riper, C. 1971. The Nature of Stuttering. Prentice-Hall, Englewood Cliffs, N.J.

Van Riper, C. 1982. The Nature of Stuttering. 2nd Ed. Prentice-Hall, Englewood Cliffs, N.J.

Wall, M. 1980. A comparison of syntax in young stutterers and nonstutterers. J. Fluency Disord. 5:345–352.

Weiss, D. 1964. Cluttering. Prentice-Hall, Englewood Cliffs,N.J.

Westby, C. 1979. Language performance of stuttering and nonstuttering children. J. Commun. Disord. 12:133–145.

Williams, D. 1978. The problem of stuttering. In: F. Darley and D. Spriestersbach (eds.), Diagnostic Methods in Speech Pathology. 2nd Ed., pp. 284–321. Harper & Row, New York.

Williams, D., and Kent, L. 1958. Listener evaluations of speech interruptions. J. Speech Hear. Res. 1:124–131.

Williams, D., Silverman, F., and Kools, J. 1969. Disfluency behavior of elementary-school stutterers and nonstutterers: Loci of instances of disfluency. J. Speech

Hear. Res. 12:308–318.
Wingate, M. 1976. Stuttering: Theory and Treatment. John Wiley & Sons, New York.

7
A Review of Therapies

Until recently, clinical researchers have given most of their attention to developing strategies to help the adult stutterer, and therapy for the child stutterer has been the "poor relation" of stuttering therapy. The views of two clinicians, Wendell Johnson and Charles Van Riper, dominated therapy for the child stutterer until the 1970's. Johnson's influence has been preeminent in that many speech-language pathologists, in treating the young child stutterer, deal directly with the parents rather than with the child. The influence of both these scholars is still reflected in much of the therapy carried out today with preschool and school-aged stutterers, with Johnson's influence appearing to be the stronger for the preschool stutterer, and Van Riper's the stronger for the school-aged stutterer.

During the past decade several therapies have emerged for the treatment of child and adult stutterers, and various developments seem to have influenced the newer trends. For example, increasing knowledge of behavior modification techniques encouraged some clinicians to organize therapy more tightly into "programs" for both child and adult stutterers. The enlarged body of knowledge of developmental psycholinguistics, and its possible interaction with the development of fluency and the development of stuttering, has caused us to pay closer attention to the "language" aspects of stuttering.

Associated with this recent knowledge are clinical observations that fluency can be influenced to a large extent by manipulations of the size and complexity of linguistic units, hence the development of language-based therapies. And finally, speech-language pathologists who want to help children of all ages to overcome stuttering have made their needs known at professional conferences where information is shared. As a result of these factors, more therapies emerged and clinicians now have choices among several more therapies than were available previously.

A frame of reference is needed for organizing a discussion of therapy approaches. A theoretical framework is not entirely satisfactory because many therapies are, at least in part, empirically based. Johnson's therapy was clearly based on his own theory of stuttering (Johnson, 1955; Johnson and Associates, 1959), but the relation between theory and therapy is not always as apparent. For convenience, therefore, this chapter is divided into two main sections—therapy for the preschool stutterer, whose age is approximately 3 to 6 years, and therapy for the school-aged stutterer, whose age is roughly 7 years to the mid-teens. A further practical, although somewhat arbitrary, subdivision is made for therapy for the preschool stutterer: therapies primarily for the parents, therapies primarily for the child, and therapies for parents and children. All therapies cannot be presented because of space limitations, nor can all details of therapies be presented. Thus the salient points of representative therapies are given, in approximate chronological order. Clinicians are encouraged to go to the original sources for further details.

THERAPIES FOR THE PRESCHOOL STUTTERER

Speech-language pathologists generally agree that young, preschool stutterers should be treated somewhat differently from older children who stutter. The thinking suggests that older children are capable of responding to direct techniques of speech management, whereas younger children are not. Clinicians continue to fear that a youngster's stuttering may be worsened by direct attention to speech, a notion that is opposed by Cooper (1979), Ryan (1979), and Shine (1980). Nevertheless, such fear has strong foundations in our professional history, and has led to the development of indirect techniques in attempts to alleviate the stuttering symptoms. The indirect approaches usually involve working with the parents through counseling rather than working with the child. If the child is also seen by the clinician for indirect therapy, the therapy would be a form of play therapy, without direct attention to speech production. Inexperienced clinicians, and those not so inexperienced, may have difficulty in deciding how to approach the young stutterer: whether to be direct or indirect, whether to treat the child or the parents, or both. The range of viewpoints presented next includes those of Johnson and Van Riper, to ensure a broad perspective.

Therapies Primarily for the Parents

Wendell Johnson   Johnson's theoretical position with the diagnosogenic theory of stuttering and later, the interaction hypothesis (Johnson and Associates, 1959), resulted in a focus on parental counseling as the sole therapy for the young stutterer. Although this position has been modified over the years, and opposing points of view have arisen, some clinicians still adhere to Johnson's theory of parent therapy as the preferred method of dealing with early stuttering.

Johnson described the beginning stutterer, for whom such therapy was developed, as follows:

> *The child may or may not be more disfluent than most children of his age. Usually, he is not apparently aware of any difference and seems to be in no sense bothered by the way he speaks. If he appears conscious of his speech in any relevant way, the evidence of it is likely to be fleeting and generally superficial. Even if, at times, he*

reacts with definitely noticeable strain and uneasiness when hesitating in speaking, most of the time he does not do this
(Johnson, 1967, p. 322).

In his counseling, Johnson sought to alleviate the parents' anxiety regarding the child's disfluencies by educating them about normal speech development, about the wide range of fluency characteristics in individuals of all ages, and about the effects of situational variation on fluency. He had the parents observe situational cues responsible for fluency breakdown in their child and suggested modifying environmental circumstances to reduce the opportunity for such breakdown. For example, Johnson thought that the following environmental situations might induce disfluency in young children: attempting to talk in too advanced a manner, such as attempting to explain things the child does not understand; speaking to an unresponsive listener; speaking in competition with others; speaking when there is conflict in the situation; speaking in circumstances that are exciting, fatiguing, bewildering, or confusing; and speaking in situations involving an impaired or insecure parent-child relationship. The range of coverage of Johnson's counseling reflects his awareness that the child may be in danger of becoming a confirmed stutterer. His reference to the child "attempting to talk in too advanced a manner" looks very much like a precursor to the recent interest in linguistic aspects of stuttering. The remainder of the situations he cites as possible cues for fluency breakdown have acted as a model, along with Van Riper's counseling, for techniques that are used today by clinicians to help the parents of young stutterers.

The point at which many, but by no means all, clinicians part company with Johnson, is the latter's belief that the parents of beginning stutterers are overly concerned about their child's fluency specifically and about speech performance generally. He thought it important to counsel the parents about "their excessive psychological need to have their child speak extremely well and perhaps to excel in other ways too and, in general, their specific discontents and their reasons for them" (Johnson, 1967, p. 326). He encouraged parents to accept their child's speech (and nonspeech) efforts and to allow the child to enjoy communication without reacting to disfluency in any way. In the article, "An Open Letter to the Mother of a Stuttering Child," Johnson (1949) advised parents to reevaluate diagnoses of their children's disfluencies as "stuttering," and he counseled them according to the points outlined above. The "letter" was widely distributed and used in this country and abroad.

In the years since Johnson expressed his views, further research has enlightened us on early childhood stuttering. We know, for example, that many children experience a spontaneous remission of stuttering (see review by Andrews et al., 1983) without therapeutic intervention. We also know that this remission may occur even in homes where the parents have asked their disfluent children to "slow down," "take a deep breath before speaking," or "stop and start over" (Cooper, 1979; Wingate, 1976). "Obviously, the old admonition that parents must not draw attention to the child's speech should be reexamined" (Cooper, 1979, p. 64). In addition, genetic studies (Andrews and Harris, 1964; Kidd, 1980) support an inherited component to stuttering in many individuals, although environmental factors are still assumed to play a role. The effect of this research is to relieve parents of the burden of necessarily being the causative agents in their child's stuttering, and this in turn affects the way in which we deal with parents in therapy. Johnson, in his writing, appears to have been sympathetic to parents, and in fact makes a plea for the clinician to understand parents as well as children (Johnson, 1967, p. 328). Nevertheless, some clinicians have created feelings of guilt in parents because of their apparent "role" in the stuttering problem of their child. Cooper (1979) and Wingate (1976) object to this approach, as do the present authors.

Johnson's advice to parents of young stutterers—to be good listeners, to reduce fluency disrupters, to understand the sequences of language and speech development, and not to be overly demanding of the child's linguistic skills—has held up over the years. However, the implied notion that the parents "caused" the stuttering has lost a lot of credence in light of newer information.

Harold Luper and Robert Mulder   Luper and Mulder (1964) divided their descriptions of therapy into four phases, to coincide with Bloodstein's four phases of the development of stuttering (Bloodstein, 1960a, 1960b, 1961, 1981). They refer to Phase 1 as *incipient* stuttering, Phase 2 as *transitional* stuttering, Phase 3 as *confirmed* stuttering, and Phase 4 as *advanced* stuttering.

Incipient stuttering is the most appropriate to include in our preschool section; it involves primarily syllable and word repetitions that are inconsistently present, lack of awareness of the disfluencies, and evaluation of the disfluencies caused by environmental pressures. Luper and Mulder also noted that hard contacts or tonic blocks may be present in children who are beginning to stutter.

Therapy aims to prevent the stuttering from developing into a more severe form, and to help the child perceive speech as being easy and pleasant. It views direct attention to the child's speech as counterproductive in that the child might, as a result, develop the perception that speech is difficult. Luper and Mulder's approach, therefore, does not deal with the child but with the environment, in particular the parents of the young stutterer.

The authors are particularly helpful when they direct their attention to the parents, and ways in which the clinician might work with them. They address areas such as parental guilt and/or anxiety, which might limit the parents' ability to use information constructively, and the constructive, as well as potentially adverse, effects of parental concern. They discuss the clinician and authority, and the tempering of "clinical authority" by the qualities of maturity, sincerity, and knowledge of one's field. Effective ways of dealing with resistance in parents are presented, as are pointers on how to handle adjustment problems or family problems that are not speech related: when to refer to other resources, how to decide between direct or indirect therapy, and how direct to be.

A series of checklists is presented, designed for the parents to work with at home and to involve them more in the therapy. One list, for example, has the parents note each time the child is given advice on how to talk, each time his stuttering is discussed in front of him, and each time someone refers to the child's speech as "stuttering" or "stammering."

Criteria for dismissal from therapy are as follows: the adults in the environment must show awareness of the roles of fear, tension, and perfectionism in stuttering, and must understand the preventive aspects of therapy; communicative pressures must be recognized and modified; an ameliorative emotional climate must be established; environmental reactions to disfluencies must no longer increase the child's awareness of disfluencies; and a satisfactory decrease in the number and severity of disfluencies must occur.

The bibliotherapy section of Luper and Mulder's therapy for the incipient stutterer is necessarily out of date. Their advice on parent counseling techniques remains pertinent, however, and may be helpful in an area where most students and many clinicians feel a deficit.

Michael Andronico and Irwin Blake   Filial therapy (Guerney, 1964), an approach of training parents to conduct nondirective play sessions with their children, was originally developed for emotionally disturbed children. However, as Andronico and Blake (1971) indicated, this psychotherapeutic approach might be beneficial for facilitating a healthier and more positive emotional atmosphere in the home for young stutterers who are also experiencing some interpersonal difficulties with their parents, or some conflict within themselves.

The basic paradigm of filial therapy includes spending the first set of sessions explaining, teaching, and illustrating to a small group of parents the techniques of nondirective play therapy. The nondirective play sessions revolve around a prescribed set of toys that have been found to promote expressions of feelings, whether such feelings are conveyed through the children's actions with the toys or through their verbalizations. The overriding emphasis of the sessions is to allow children to express themselves freely (with minimal restraints except, for instance, that they cannot physically harm the parents) and, equally important, to cultivate in the parents a manner of responding to and interacting with their children that conveys acceptance and empathy by being "in tune" with their children's feelings.

The parents continue to meet in the weekly group sessions, but they also begin play therapy sessions at home once they are comfortable with the techniques and once the clinicians, who are presumably well trained in the techniques themselves, feel that the parents are competent to conduct the play therapy. A major tool used during these sessions is reflective listening, modeled after Rogerian counseling. A note of caution should be sounded in the use of filial therapy—that is, the clinician should have conducted nondirective play therapy under close supervision before attempting to train parents in using the techniques. A byproduct of the weekly parent group sessions is the expression of many interpersonal and emotional conflicts parents experience with their child, regardless of whether these problems are associated with the child's stuttering. Although filial therapy does not by itself deal directly with the child's fluency behavior, Andronico and Blake conjecture and, indeed, have observed that a reduced rate of stuttering may ensue after the sessions, in part because the parents convey acceptance of the child as a whole rather than focusing solely on the negative symptoms of stuttering.

Oliver Bloodstein   According to Bloodstein (1981), most therapy for early childhood stuttering emphasizes parent counseling, perhaps accompanied by play therapy for the child. He sees this in part as stemming from Johnson's diagnosogenic theory, and in part from Van Riper's emphasis on the dichotomy of primary and secondary stuttering, in which primary stuttering is viewed as an earlier and much simpler phenomenon than secondary stuttering (Bluemel, 1932, 1957; Van Riper, 1963). Bloodstein also assesses the prevailing viewpoint of early stuttering as that of an emotional disorder of childhood, with parent counseling thus the preferred method of treatment.

Essentially Bloodstein's advice to parents parallels that of Wendell Johnson. Parents and significant others in the environment are requested not to criticize or intervene in any negative way with the child's speech. Counseling seeks to reduce perfectionism of the parents with regard to the child. Speaking situations for the youngster are made more pleasant, with a reduction in pressure situations such as speaking in competition with others and oral confessions of guilt. Rather, the parents are encouraged to provide successful speaking situations for the child where fluency will more likely occur, as in choral speaking, rhythmic speaking, and reciting nursery rhymes. In addition, Bloodstein suggests a reduction in the rate of speech and complexity of vocabulary of the parents, a notion that has been reflected in the approaches of other clinicians.

Linda J. Johnson   A contrasting method of working with early childhood stutterers through their parents is presented by L. J. Johnson (1980), who places therapy in the theoretical frameworks of discoordination and operant conditioning. Johnson teaches the parents of young stutterers to speak at a slowed speech rate to provide a model for the children that will promote smooth, coordinated, and integrated speech attempts. In addition, using the rationale that the children may learn the "manipulative value of disfluency," she has the parents selectively attend to their children's speech so that they respond only to the fluent utterances. Theoretically this technique should result in the reinforcement of fluency and the nonreinforcement (and therefore reduction) of disfluent utterances. Parents are trained to keep daily logs of their work with the children. Logs and weekly audiotapes are reviewed by parents and clinician at biweekly sessions. Counseling on general management problems with the children is provided as needed, but is secondary to the home program for stuttering.

Johnson reports on seven children who received such therapy, for an average length of 4 months. Children and parents were discharged when the clinician felt the parents were capable of using the program independently and when the child's disfluencies were decreasing. Most followup evaluations were made by telephone contact with the parents, and by analysis of an audiotape sent to the clinician. Five of the seven children progressed to being normally fluent; one achieved reasonable fluency but regressed after a change in environment; the seventh was unavailable for reevaluation.

Therapies Primarily for the Child

The therapies included in this section spell out in detail therapy for the young child. These approaches do not, however, preclude parent counseling when it is indicated (Ryan, 1979; Stocker, 1980).

Bruce Ryan   Ryan (1971, 1979) has made a concerted attempt to organize therapy procedures so that each phase of therapy is carefully detailed, resulting in a series of steps based on learning theory that, he feels, any speech-language pathologist can follow. His use of the operant principles of stimulus control and contingency management led to programs in which over many small, consecutive steps, successive approximation procedures shape fluency to the final goal of fluent conversation. Before starting the therapy, base rates of stuttering are obtained (percentage of stuttering and stuttered words per minute—SW/M), and a rate measurement is made (words spoken per minute—WS/M). The base rates are established for tasks of reading (for the older child), monologue, and conversation. The client must exhibit more than 0.5 SW/M to begin therapy.

The overall program of fluency shaping consists of establishment, transfer, and maintenance phases of therapy. First comes the *establishment* of fluency in the client's spontaneous speech in controlled conditions, or in the clinical situation. Then that fluency is *transferred* into other situations, such as the home and the school of the stutterer. Finally the fluency must be *maintained* in life situations on a long-term basis.

Ryan sets criterion levels for each stage of the program. A client who does not reach criterion level is recycled through the entire program, or part of it. Branching steps exist for those requiring additional work at specific levels. In earlier work with children Ryan (1971) reported using verbal reinforcers such as "good" and "that's right"; in one case, points, which could be exchanged for release time from therapy, were the reward. In the packaged kit by Ryan and Van Kirk (1978), reinforcement is speci-fied as "social" or "redeemable tokens" and the schedule of reinforcement is described.

Two programs have evolved from the clinical research of Ryan (1971, 1979) and Ryan and Van Kirk (1974)—delayed auditory feedback (DAF) and gradual increase in length and complexity of utterance (GILCU). The DAF program incorporates reading and is said to be preferable for the older or the more severe stutterer, although Ryan has used it on a client as young as 7 years (Ryan, 1971). The GILCU is said to be more efficient with the younger or the less severe stutterer. Ryan reported using this method on children as young as 4 years of age. The establishment phases of therapy differ for the DAF and GILCU programs, but the transfer and maintenance phases remain the same.

The GILCU, as stated, is advised for young children and for mild to moderate stutterers. A reading section of the program is optional. The client begins by reading (or, if a nonreader, naming or imitating) one-word utterances fluently, then two-word utterances, and then up to six-word utterances. Sentences are introduced and the client is required to remain fluent on one sentence, two sentences, and so on up to four sentences. Fluent monologues are introduced beginning at 30 seconds long and grad-ually increasing the time to 5 minutes.

The transfer program uses variation of the physical setting, audience size, speaking to strangers (or less familiar people), use of the telephone, and using fluency in the home and at school if appropriate. If the client fails to maintain fluency, he is recycled through the necessary steps of the program. A successfully treated child is one who achieves 0.5 SW/M or less.

Ryan (1979) reported that an average of 20 to 30 hours of clinician time is required over a 2-year period to complete the therapy and that the success rate using this and other programs with children has been high. Specifically related to the GILCU program are the results of therapy on 14 children aged 4 to 8 years. Pretherapy SW/M was 11.8 and posttherapy SW/M was 0.2. Regarding followup, Ryan comments that most clients who have become fluent in the programs have retained fluency.

Richard Shine   Shine's approach to the treatment of young stutterers is also very direct, and bears some similarities to Ryan's GILCU (Shine, 1980). Shine controls the length and complexity of utterance of the children, gradually increasing the demands of linguistic complexity and motor planning required for the utterance. An "easy speaking voice" is encouraged. Using a token system of reward, Shine outlines five steps of fluency training: 1) a picture identification task in which the child names familiar pictures, retaining fluency; 2) development of speaking variables that will enhance fluency, such as whispered speech for naming, which is gradually shaped toward spontaneous, voiced phrase production; 3) fluency training during highly structured activities, from picture naming (monosyllabic words to multisyllabic words) to story book descriptions and language games; 4) fluency training during conversational speech and generalization to other speech environments, using transfer activities as required; and 5) maintenance of fluency that involves gradual decrease in therapy for at least a year. Conversational speech in which the children might stutter is discouraged in the early stages of fluency training, unless the child adopts a way of speaking, such as whispering, that results in fluency.

Although Shine's focus in therapy is the child, the parents are involved in the treatment process. They are taught to identify, count, and tally stutterings, and are encouraged to adopt a slower rate of speech. Like Ryan, Shine's criterion of success is 0.5 or fewer SW/M. He reports that 17 of 20 children were discharged as fluent, and that average treatment time was 10.4 months.

Beatrice Stocker   The Stocker probe technique is designed to differentiate normally nonfluent youngsters from young stutterers, and to provide a fluency-shaping program for children as young as 3 years; no upper age limit is given (Stocker, 1980). The probes are questions or requests that elicit information from the child. Basic to the rationale of the probes is Stocker's belief that "increasing levels of demand" applied to the child incur increasing quantities of stuttering. "Level of demand" is equated with "communicative responsibility." On Level I, the child is asked to respond to an either/or question, whereas on Level V he or she is requested to make up a story about an object. According to Stocker, "As we ascend these levels, the disfluent child stutters more. There is a strong correlation between the demand for creativity and the effect on fluency; and as we ascend these levels, demands for creativity are higher" (Stocker, 1980, p. 11).

The overall program consists of five steps: the initial evaluation, establishing a baseline, achieving therapy goals, carrying out ongoing evaluations, and reevaluation of the child's speech. For the initial evaluation, probes are presented randomly with regard to level; therapy begins at the level below which the child first experienced disfluencies, and works through the sequence of levels from 1 to 5.

When the child is disfluent he returns to a lower level of demand as determined by the clinician, and then works forward again. He is rewarded with predetermined reinforcers (stars, praise, tokens) for fluency exceeding baseline or for three successive 60-second periods of fluency.

Therapy may begin with heightening the child's awareness of his own (or others') disfluencies, and may attend to the elimination of secondary characteristics, in addition to reinforcing fluency. Generally two 25-minute sessions per week are considered to be appropriate, although a higher frequency is recommended.

With regard to differentiating normally nonfluent children from stutterers, Stocker suggests that the former exhibit disfluency without respect to level, whereas the latter exhibit increasing disfluency as the level of demand increases. Stocker mentions the inclusion of parent counseling in the program, in addition to attending to individual needs of the clients.

Therapies for Parents and Children

Charles Van Riper   Van Riper (1973) aims to promote fluency in the young stutterer but does not work directly on speech to achieve that end. He believes, by and large, that young children (mostly preschoolers) are not aware of their stuttering; therefore he refers to these children as "beginning" stutterers. Although Van Riper desensitizes the children to impending stuttering, he does not desensitize them to situation and word fears as he would with an older stutterer, because he has not observed such symptoms in "beginning" youngsters. His therapy incorporates the use of appropriate fluency models, the facilitation of fluency, counterconditioning, reducing the stimulus value of stuttering, removing other stresses in the child's life, and parent counseling.

Several aspects of Van Riper's therapy for the beginning stutterer are worthy of discussion. For example, his program is thorough in its attempt to ensure that the child regains as well as maintains fluency. He searches out "other stresses" in the child's life and deals with them, lest they in some way act to maintain the stuttering. Parents are taught how to listen to their children, how to handle their own feelings about the stuttering, and how to encourage the child to talk on his fluent days but not on his disfluent days.

Although Van Riper does not work directly on the stuttering symptoms, he has devised methods of facilitating and reinforcing fluency. This is done partially through rhythm activities accompanying speech. Another method is to use successive approximations to get, for example, from whispered single-word utterances to loud voice words, to whispered phrases, to loud voice phrases, and finally to fluent voiced spontaneous speech.

His method of desensitizing a child to impending stuttering has been widely practiced. He plays and converses with the child, who is, in this benign situation, usually fluent. Gradually the clinician applies increasing pressure until the child shows signs of tension and imminent stuttering. At this point the clinician backs off, reducing the pressure and allowing the child to return to the former level of calm and fluency. The desensitization is then begun again. This repeated process is designed to help the child resist the threat of stuttering, to show the child that stuttering need not follow a threatening situation, and at the same time to reinforce the child's fluency.

Van Riper is extremely creative in the suggestions he gives for reinforcing fluency. Many suggestions emanate from specific cases in which he designed techniques to suit the needs of individual children. His clinicians demonstrate a firm understanding and knowledge of stuttering, an understanding that enables them to examine the phenomenon and to deal with it without fear.

Van Riper discusses a variety of therapies that focus on stuttering as a type of language disorder by aiming "to help the child to organize his speech and to help him formulate and express his thoughts" (Van Riper, 1973, p. 381). Although Van Riper does not try to specify the nature of a possible linguistic component in stuttering, he believes that the parents can be possible agents of fluency disruption by excessive linguistic demands.

> *Stuttering usually begins at the very time that great advances in sentence construction occur and it seems tenable that when the speech models provided by the parents or siblings of the child are too difficult for him to follow, some faltering will ensue*
> (Van Riper, 1973, p. 381).

This therapy is multifaceted and designed to cover all bases. It is structured insofar as the clinician has specific goals in mind, but it is carried out in a low structured setting. It requires a thorough understanding of stuttering and its ramifications, and is best handled by a clinician who is willing to be creative and to tailor therapy to the specific needs of the child and the family.

Martin Adams   Adams (1980) attempts to dovetail therapy procedures with the presenting symptoms. For example, if the child belongs to the group he calls the "motor-impaired group," and has difficulty in initiating or in sustaining voice, therapy focuses on easy onset or on sustaining voice. Some type of breath stream management is incorporated into therapy for the "motor-impaired group." The child is taught to speak more slowly with slight prolongation of speech sounds, similar to the speech pattern that stutterers use under the delayed auditory feedback (DAF) condition. ". . . the child is given specific instructions and a behavioral model to follow, so that he will adopt the prolonged speech pattern and thus produce his clinical responses at a slower rate" (Adams, 1980, p. 292). The rationale for using a slower speech rate is to simplify the timing and coordination of the motor gestures required for speech production and the way in which they synchronize with the airstream.

After the motor act of speech has been simplified Adams uses an adaptation of "gradual increase in the length and complexity of utterance" (GILCU) (Ryan, 1971, 1979; Ryan and Van Kirk, 1978; see also this chapter, under "Therapies Primarily for the Child") to transfer the newer speech pattern into increasingly long and complex language units.

Adams identifies a second group of young stutterers as the "language-impaired group." This group ". . . may have stuttering problems that derive exclusively from slowness and uncertainty in the operation of various aspects of the language encoding process (for example, word retrieval) (Adams, 1980, p. 293). Use of the rate reduction technique and Ryan's GILCU allow the child sufficient time to coordinate the complex process of communication.

Adams stresses the importance of applying procedures of operant conditioning appropriately: the response-contingent positive reinforcer must be appealing to the child; it must be given as soon as the response has been made; a 100% reinforcement schedule should be maintained for acquisition of a response, and then a variable ratio reinforcement schedule should be applied to achieve resistance to extinction.

With regard to the transfer stage of therapy, Adams reiterates what others have noted, that some young stutterers make remarkably quick and easy transfer of their new fluency to their individual environments (Adams, 1980; Ryan, 1979; Shine, 1980). However, his incorporation of the parents into the program is designed to facilitate transfer. Parents are phased into therapy when the child has attained minimal fluency. At first the parents sit far behind the child in the therapy room, and gradually they move closer, until parents, child, and clinician are around the table together. Ultimately the parents assume a clinical role, home practice is assigned, and the parents become reinforcing agents.

THERAPIES FOR THE SCHOOL-AGED STUTTERER

There seem to be several advantages to treating the school-aged stutterer. Presumably the school setting should facilitate efficient therapy because the speech-language pathologist has access to the child in an environment of situational influences that change over a period of some 6 hours each day for 5 days a week. This should surely assist the clinician in getting to know the child and the stuttering, and in helping the child to transfer gains of fluency or modification skills from the clinical office to everyday life. Not so, say many school clinicians, who frequently are too overwhelmed by large caseloads to be able to take therapeutic advantage of the situation for the child. In addition, difficulties arise: inaccessible parents, some youngsters who feel and behave like "captive clients" because they have no choice but to be in therapy, and occasional dilemmas about the child's reactions to being removed from class to attend therapy. Moreover, therapy for the school-aged stutterer has remained even less specific than for the preschooler. The summaries that follow are representative of the range of therapies currently known.

Charles Van Riper

Van Riper (1973), in his chapter "Treatment of the Young Confirmed Stutterer," gives the age range of such youngsters as about 7 to 14 years. He acknowledges a possible overlap of symptoms of the "confirmed" group with the "beginning stutterer" discussed in the section on therapies for the preschool stutterer. He emphasizes the importance of the relationship between the client and clinician. One of the reasons for this importance is that the child may need to use the clinician as a surrogate parent figure.

The broad outline of therapy is the same as that for adults, that is: identification of symptoms, desensitization, modification, and stabilization. Considerable adjustments are made, however, to accommodate the younger stutterer. In the identification stage, for example, the child stutterer usually is not as finely analytic about his blocks as the adult stutterer, but he is aware of gross instrumental acts, such as head jerks. Because struggle and escape behaviors are difficult for the child to handle directly, it is suggested that they be differentiated from easier speech by the use of the terms "hard stuttering" and "easy stuttering." Van Riper thinks that this child can deal with avoidance, postponements, and starters more easily than with the struggle and escape reactions.

The school-aged stutterer, according to Van Riper, can probably discuss his feared situations and can, with guidance from the clinician, learn to enter and cope with such situations. In addition, Van Riper recommends desensitization to speech interrupters and to other stimuli perceived as frustrating by the child.

As in therapy for the preschool child, fluency-enhancing techniques, such as rhythmic speaking, are used to reinforce fluency. At an appropriate time, Van Riper inserts easy pseudostuttering into his own speech during conversations with the child. This demonstrates to the child that it is possible to be disfluent without tension. It also provides a model for the child, who frequently begins using this easy pattern of stuttering spontaneously instead of struggling. The easier pattern of stuttering, where the child experiences slow transitions from sound to sound, is considered to be a modification of the stuttering. According to Van Riper, this type of modification is all that is necessary to reverse the course of stuttering in some children.

If necessary, further modification of the block is taught in the form of cancellation and pullouts, but not preparatory sets, for Van Riper has observed that usually the child automatically begins to assume correct preparatory sets, because there is: ". . . a natural tendency for the new way of stuttering to move forward in time, from cancellation to pullout and from that to an automatic preparatory set. This seems to occur without any formal training" (Van Riper, 1973, p. 45).

Van Riper's discussion of cancellation for adults is more than nine pages long. A succinct description has been extracted:

> . . . *once the person emits a stuttered word, he simply pauses deliberately and then says it again before going on. With all the vehemence we can muster, let us emphasize that there is much more to the cancellation process than the mere repetition of a stuttered word. Many therapists have not understood that cancellation is designed primarily as a vehicle for learning new responses to the stimuli that trigger the abnormal stuttering responses. It is a miniature learning laboratory and it's portable. We see very little value in merely saying a stuttered word again fluently*
> (Van Riper, 1973, p. 319).

That somewhat complex explanation is for the adult. Van Riper adjusted this presentation of cancellation for the school-aged child as follows:

> *If we can get the child to correct his moments of old stuttering behaviors by pausing, and then by stuttering in the new easy way, we do much to weaken the strength of the old behaviors but we must recognize that often we cannot get this correction*
> (Van Riper, 1973, p. 442).

The cautionary note is sounded because children often are in a hurry to communicate and find cancellation very difficult to accomplish. Van Riper's pullout is designed essentially to have the stutterer ease the tension in the block and gradually coarticulate with the rest of the word.

Stabilization is thought to be easier with the school-aged child than with the adult. In addition to the more direct aspects of his therapy, Van Riper includes parent counseling in the overall plan and attends to any significant areas of the environment. Parents observe therapy and are helped to develop the capacity to deal openly with the stuttering.

Dean Williams

Williams (1971) pointed out that therapy for the school-aged stutterer is frequently a form of adult therapy. He suggests that the school clinician give special attention to characteristics that might be unique to the younger, although not the *very* young, age group. For example, school-aged children may not be as aware of sound/word difficulties associated with their stuttering as adult stutterers, but Williams's impression is that the clinician may help the stutterer over time to detect and work on such difficulties. Similarly, the school-aged stutterer may not be prepared to discuss reactions and feelings. In spite of this, Williams advocates discussion with the child, and a seemingly psychotherapeutic milieu is suggested. Discussion with the child might center on, for example, learning to make mistakes, learning to accept feelings, and learning new nonspeech behavior.

Williams is enthusiastic about school as the ideal setting for therapy because he supports Johnson's interaction hypothesis, which postulates a disturbed interaction between the stutterer and the people in his environment. At school the clinician is in a position to observe interactions and to handle them therapeutically. For example, if the client's teacher reacts to the child holding his breath during speech, that behavior (breath holding) is worked on early in therapy, so that the interaction between the teacher and the child can be more positive. If the parents perceive certain adjustment problems (such as an overly messy room), they are helped to cope with the situations.

The most direct therapy that Williams mentions is that the child learns to talk easily in therapy. Role playing follows, with the clinician assuming roles of the significant people in the child's environment and the child continuing to talk easily throughout the change of roles. Stutterers are requested to use "easy speech" instead of "hard speech," and parents and teachers are requested to reinforce easy speech.

In later writing, Williams (1979) emphasized three aspects of therapy for the school-aged stutterer. First, the child is guided to explore the possible influence of emotional reactions on the degree of tension in speech production. Second, the child needs to become attuned to the natural behavioral process of nonspeech body movement, and the process of its disruption. Finally, easy, forward-moving speech must be emphasized. These therapy goals are integrated, and with discussion are incorporated into practice sessions of behavior changes.

Harold Luper and Robert Mulder

Having dealt with Luper and Mulder's incipient stutterer in the preschool therapy section of this chapter, we consider their transitional, confirmed, and advanced stutterers with the school-aged clients (Luper and Mulder, 1964). Transitional stuttering is chronic, but fluctuates in severity. Some children are susceptible to situational influences on stuttering, and excitement is probably the predominant situational cue. Children at this stage may call themselves stutterers, but they speak freely and demonstrate little concern about the condition. As for the incipient stutterer, the transitional stutterer may receive indirect therapy only, by virtue of the clinician working through the environment. The child may, however, have face-to-face therapy with the clinician, which may focus on direct speech production even though the child's attention is not drawn directly to his stuttering.

Parent counseling at this stage of development will be similar to that for the incipient stutterer. Luper and Mulder make a nice point when they discuss the parent who may need help in moving from an attitude of "unconcern" or "ignoring" the stuttering, to a more constructive attitude toward the child. The parents may be deeply concerned, perhaps experiencing considerable inner turmoil, while ostensibly ignoring the condition. The child may be in a state of confusion, knowing that there is a difficulty in talking, yet filled with uncertainty because no one else seems to think so. A calm, uncomplicated acknowledgment of the problem by the parents to the child is suggested.

As for direct attention to the speech, Van Riper's desensitization procedures (Van Riper, 1973) are used to help to prepare the child to participate in our "talking society," and the technique of loose contacts is taught to the child if applicable. (See Chapter 8, p. 196, for discussion of "loose contacts.")

Less direct ways of strengthening fluency include: 1) providing the child with opportunities to talk successfully, 2) encouraging as much participation in oral class and school activities as the child can manage, 3) giving the child the chance to participate in choral activities, 4) attending to any nonspeech areas that need attention, such as hearing or vision, and 5) reinforcing the child's strengths and giving due praise.

Luper and Mulder state that the symptoms of confirmed stutterers are "full-fledged." Word and situational avoidance is present but not habitual. Secondary characteristics are appearing; the child is aware of the stuttering and requires direct help. The ages of this group range from as young as 8 years to adulthood.

Objectives for the initial therapy period are: 1) helping the child to understand the nature of his therapy goals, such as modification of attitude and of speech behavior, 2) helping the child to develop realistic personal goals for self-help, 3) helping the stutterer to be less sensitive about stuttering, and 4) developing a healthy clinical relationship with the child.

Luper and Mulder suggest caution with regard to working on non-avoidance techniques and development of the "objective attitude" with a stutterer at this stage of development. ". . . the reduction of fear is probably accomplished more easily and less dangerously by providing successful speaking situations than it is by direct discussions and strong urging to enter feared situations" (Luper and Mulder, 1964, p. 113). In the 1960's, "objective attitude" referred to a therapy technique that required the stutterer to openly discuss his stuttering with family, friends, and even total strangers.

Direct attempts to modify the stuttering begin by eliciting from the child descriptions of what he or she did at the time of speech breakdown, and how it was done. The clinician encourages the child to notice the ways in which stuttering occurred on words, although not on all stuttered words. This is considered to be the beginning stage of a sense of control.

Even more direct attempts to modify the stuttering are then attempted with the use of loose contacts, cancellation, and pullouts. Luper and Mulder give useful analogies of all these techniques, so that the child may visualize the technique (in a form involving, e.g., an athletic event) before attempting it in speech. Luper and Mulder regard loose contacts as an extremely valuable technique that sometimes results in markedly reduced tension and, as a result, fear reduction also. Further symptom work is directed to ensuring that the child uses appropriate phonetic placements at the onsets of words. Such articulatory contacts are to be appropriate and relaxed, then moving to an easy transition to the next sound. By this time, the stutterer also has learned to manage the associated symptoms. In addition to these direct techniques, the child needs help in eliminating the fears of specific words, and of situations.

The symptoms of advanced stuttering include strong anticipation of stuttering, distress on the part of the child, and fully developed symptoms with a wide range of secondary characteristics and emotional reactions of fear and embarrassment. The authors stress the seriousness of the disorder when the stutterer has reached this advanced stage, and feel that such a child may be in severe emotional distress.

An objective attitude is important in therapy for the advanced stutterer, according to Luper and Mulder. Two changes that the child is encouraged to make in becoming "more accepting and less emotional about what he does" are as follows: to be willing to allow others to know about the stuttering and resist the temptation to hide or minimize it, and to be willing to enter difficult speaking situations even if expecting to stutter. As an advanced stutterer, the child is to accept responsibility for working on his or her speech, whereas in the earlier stages the responsibility was taken largely by the clinician and parents.

Luper and Mulder are at their best in offering nondirective counseling techniques to the clinician. They suggest ways to elicit information from the client so that the information sharing reveals details of the stuttering to the stutterer. Within the framework of the semantic therapy proposed by Johnson (1946) and Williams (1957), the child is encouraged to describe what happens during talking, rather than what happens to him or to her (the latter implying no control). For example:

> *Instead of "my lips wouldn't open" he is encouraged to report that he held his lips pressed tightly together. Instead of "my tongue was stuck" he describes his actions in terms of "I jammed my tongue against my upper teeth" or "I didn't move my tongue"*
> (Luper and Mulder, 1964, p. 157).

The client is also encouraged to allow the stuttering to emerge, to drop some avoidances and do the feared thing (i.e., stuttering), to accept any consequences of the stuttering, and ultimately to control the stuttering as it emerges. The child must strive for a change of response to speech cues so that there is a reduction of anxiety in anticipation of speech and consequent lack of tension, and finally a lack of or reduction of stuttering. The stutterer is taught to modify the symptom through the use of cancellation, pullouts, and preparatory sets.

Assignments are recommended as a means of making therapy more concrete and having the child take responsibility for therapy. The need for positive reinforcement for accomplishments of the client is stressed. Luper and Mulder give criteria for discharge from therapy at each level of stuttering.

James Frick

Frick's motor planning therapy (Frick, 1970) seems to be suitable for the school-aged stutterer, although he does not make this specific claim. Basic to the therapy is Frick's belief that stutterers stutter because they are unable to plan the sequence of motor acts required for speech. The stutterer may, for example, assume an unnatural articulatory posture in "getting ready" for an utterance, then be unable to move from that posture into the overlapping sequential movements that are essential for speech. According to Frick, the lack of motor planning that characterizes the speech breakdown is likely to take place when the stutterer is in a fearful situation and/or when anticipating stuttering. Frick employs techniques designed to improve the stutterer's ability to plan speech motorically, as well as direct techniques for modification of the block and attention to the stutterer's attitude and self-concept as needed. The four techniques used for motor planning are structuring, developing awareness of breakdown in motor planning, becoming aware of fluency, and improving motor planning ability.

Structuring is the sharing of information about motor planning with the client. Frick uses analogies from sports and dance to illustrate the fluid, sequential movements that result from motor planning for any skilled movement, speech or otherwise. Although motor planning for speech is an unconscious activity, for the stutterer it will need to become more conscious, as the next phase of therapy demonstrates.

As part of the task in developing an awareness of the breakdown in motor planning, the client is asked to evaluate expectations of stuttering immediately before answering a question posed by the clinician. More specifically, the stutterer determines whether stuttering is expected. If it is expected, the client determines the nature of the awareness—kinesthetic, auditory, or visual cues. The same self-appraisal occurs during silent reading, whenever the client expects to stutter on a word.

Next, the stutterer's awareness of fluency is heightened by feeling the movements of fluency, and viewing them in a mirror. Awareness of fluency is also heightened by the use of the tape recorder, as in listening to tape-recorded segments of his or her fluent utterances, then perhaps repeating them fluently. Fluency as a "feeling of ongoingness and motion" is stressed in activities such as the examples cited.

In attempting to improve the client's motor planning ability, there is an effort to establish "the habit of fluent thinking." In this task the client responds to a question first by thinking the responses, then by signaling the clinician that the fluency of the answer is acceptable, and finally by uttering the response. The procedure of fluency is repeated if necessary. Frick states that ". . . the procedure is an attempt to train the stutterer to develop a voluntary conscious motor plan of non-stuttering speech" (Frick, 1970, p. 14). Other techniques suggested to improve planning ability include conscious attention to motor planning while repeating a stuttered word until it is fluent, or repeating a phrase containing the stuttered word until it is fluent.

In addition to the therapy procedures above, Frick teaches a form of Van Riper's cancellation technique to the stutterer. Instead of the cancellation taking place immediately after the stuttered word, it takes place after completion of the phrase. This is because Frick believes that the motor planning for speech takes place for phrase-length units rather than word-length units. Suggestions are also made for helping the client to incorporate gains in fluency into spontaneous speech.

Eugene Cooper

Cooper's method of dealing directly with stuttering in children is through a technique he refers to as "FIGs" (fluency-initiating gestures) and a graphic representation called the "stuttering apple" (Cooper, 1965, 1979), which he states can be used with very young children. Because of some focus on introspection and examination of feelings and reactions, however, Cooper's approach is placed with therapies for the older child stutterer.

Maintaining that the FIGs seem to be effective in eliciting fluency in children, Cooper makes the task more tangible to the children by having them draw a FIG tree, with some large figs, in which the children write their own FIGs that are useful to them (or place meaningful symbols, if not writers).

The "stuttering apple" is also a visual representation of the child's speech production, symbolizing the difficulties experienced rather than the methods for coping with them. The core of the apple is drawn on paper; this represents blocking on a word and may be described as "getting stuck" or whatever term has been used with the child. The clinician draws a circle around and attached to the core of the apple each time the child identifies a characteristic of symptomatology, such as blinking the eyes or avoiding speech. That is, the stuttering symptoms are all components of the "stuttering apple." In choosing an achievable goal from the apple to begin work on with the youngster, Cooper feels that therapy becomes more concrete for the child rather than remaining abstract.

When the child can use FIGs effectively, the "feeling of fluency control" is the next goal. Cooper describes this feeling in part by stating that: "It is the visceral response of knowing you are capable of controlling a complex motor act" (1979, p. 82). A stutterer who has the "feeling of control" should be able to exert control over the stuttering (and fluency) by using his FIGs.

Cooper has developed four stages of a personalized fluency control therapy, which incorporates the FIGs. The stages of therapy are identification and structuring, examination and confrontation, cognition and behavior orientation, and fluency control.

According to Cooper, the interaction or rapport between clinician and client is extremely important to the effectiveness of therapy because feelings and attitudes of the stutterer must be dealt with. Indeed, some aspects of the personalized fluency control therapy appear to be rather adult oriented in their focus on self-evaluation and confrontation. On a more practical note, Cooper provides a variety of checklists and ratings for use by clinicians with clients and parents.

Donald Mowrer

Mowrer (1979) developed his "program to establish fluent speech" based on learning theory principles and therefore using behavior modification techniques. It is designed for children (and adults) who can read minimally at a second-grade level and is an establishment program only; there are no transfer and maintenance phases of therapy.

Mowrer bases the structure of the program on the word-bound grammatical studies of Brown (1945) and the study by Eisenson and Horowitz (1945) that suggested a relation between stuttering and the propositionality of language. As a result Mowrer has devised lists of stimulus words that in the early stages begin more frequently with vowels than with consonants, and words that are more likely to be function words (articles, prepositions, conjunctions, pronouns) than content words (nouns, adverbs, adjectives, verbs). The word lists change gradually to incorporate stimuli that are believed to be more substantive and to induce more stuttering, and the linguistic units required of the stutterer become longer. The size of the units increases from one word to two, to three-word phrases, to sentences of increasing length, and then to stories.

The rate of the client's speech is paced by a tape recording of beeps that occur every 5 seconds and serve to establish a slow rate of speech. The client is advised to skip any words that may produce stuttering. The beeped signal is gradually faded and eliminated. No advice is given to the stutterers on how to handle or manage blocking. However, a monotone voice is used at first to promote fluency. In addition, tasks are repeated so that through adaptation, more fluency will occur.

Criterion levels are given for each of the steps in the five sections of the program, with suggested branching steps if the client cannot reach criterion level. Reinforcement ratios are specified, and verbal praise or rewards are used as reinforcers.

The final goal of the program is to converse with the clinician about selected topics for 5 minutes, still using a variable ratio of reinforcement, and with the client maintaining 98% fluency. The estimated length of therapy time is 8 to 10 hours.

Bruce Ryan and Barbara Van Kirk

Ryan and Van Kirk (1974) documented their DAF program for adults and have included the DAF program in their therapy for children (1978). They report having used it on a child as young as 7 years.

The therapy begins with binaural presentation of DAF at a 250-msec delay, and the client is instructed to read with a slow, prolonged speech pattern. The amount of delay is gradually reduced to 200, 150, 100, and 50 msec, then 50-msec delay monaurally, and finally fluent reading without delay. A similar paradigm is repeated for monologue and conversational speech. The rate control program follows the DAF program and is designed to get the client's speech rate within normal limits for reading, monologue, and conversation.

Transfer and maintenance are the same as for the GILCU program described earlier in this chapter.

Carl Dell

Dell (1980) has devoted his writing exclusively to the school-aged stutterer in an effort to assist school clinicians in their planning of therapy. For convenience, he addresses the borderline stutterer, the mild stutterer, and the confirmed stutterer, as well as ways of working with parents and with teachers. His approach is Van Riperian in that he seeks to help the stutterer to acknowledge and to identify stuttering, and eventually to modify it in the direction of fluency. The goal appears to be easier stuttering rather than fluency per se. The stutterer is encouraged to pay increasingly refined attention to the stuttering block, to be able to identify or to specify where in the vocal tract the blockage is occurring. Desensitization procedures are incorporated into therapy, at first to help the child tolerate stuttering in others and later as a method of building control over "easy speech" during role playing involving authority figures. Various techniques are presented to help the stutterers get control over the block: deliberate prolongation of a sound that is terminated at a predetermined signal, pseudostuttering, and cancellation.

In dealing with a child who seems unsure of the reason for therapy, Dell suggests a direct, but kind, confrontational approach, such as: "I'm the speech teacher and I help children who sometimes have trouble talking. How about you? Do you have trouble talking?" (Dell, 1980, p. 23).

The presentations of dialogue between clinician and child may be very helpful to the inexperienced clinician. On the whole, Dell suggests an attitude of casual curiosity about the stuttering on the part of the clinician because he has found this effective in eliciting cooperation from the child. He encourages sensitivity to the child's needs and an empathetic response to the "low points" of therapy.

Ronald Webster

The Precision Fluency Shaping Program: Speech Reconstruction for Stutterers (Webster, 1979) is a standardized therapy for stutterers that sets out a series of target steps to be followed sequentially. The program was designed for, and has been used primarily with, adults, but Webster states that it has been used effectively with children aged 5 to 12 years.

The program is an intensive one in which the stutterer works for 19 days to achieve fluency, clocking about 100 hours of fluent speech in that time. Speech tasks are broken down into target behaviors beginning with the production of fluent sounds and syllables. Each target is "operationally defined" and based on knowledge of the physiology of respiration, phonation, and articulation for speech. A voice monitor, a device sensitive to intensity rise time, gives visual feedback if phonation or speech is initiated easily. The targets, which are the primary component of the program, are carefully sequenced. They are practiced repeatedly until they are "over-learned," with the initial fluent sounds and syllables being incorporated ultimately into longer utterances.

The transfer of targets is begun quite early in the program by using a limited number of targets outside the clinic. With the client's increasing control over the speech units, the transfer activities become more complex and intense. Transfer activities include telephone calls (at least 100), making speeches in front of other clients, and speaking in stores and local businesses.

In taking pre- and posttherapy base rates of stuttering, Webster counts all disfluencies, even phrase repetitions. A normal range of fluency is achieved when the disfluencies are below 3%, and they are brief and effortless.

In contrast to many therapies for stutterers, Webster does not include desensitization. "We are discovering that when the client has achieved control over fluency-generating targets, he can normally speak fluently in spite of fears, anxieties and life stresses" (Webster, 1979, p. 220). Accessory features are said to subside, not requiring special attention. The program is not adjusted for "individual needs" of clients, although some may spend more time on the various steps than others. This therapy is available only by attending Webster's facility or that of a clinician who has been trained by Webster. The treatment program is not available commercially.

DISCUSSION

Most clinicians whose points of view and therapies are described in this chapter give the impression, in their original works, that they are reasonably content with the results of their therapy with young stutterers. They seem to be generally optimistic about therapy for the preschool child, regardless of whether they present data to support their successes. That does not appear to be the case with regard to the school-aged stutterers, where even fewer data are presented. The child who can no longer participate on the naive level of the preschooler, and who has not yet developed the motivated and objective outlook of the adult, seems to remain something of an enigma to clinicians. Van Riper has resolved this by finding ways to enter the child's world, so that he can then lead the child toward changing the stuttering pattern. Ryan's program stays outside the child's feelings, precisely organizing the stimuli designed to bring speech closer and closer to normally fluent conversation. The earlier focus on modification of the stuttering has given way, to some extent, to an interest in attempting to achieve fluency through fluency-shaping procedures, or an integrated version of these approaches (Guitar and Peters, 1980).

Clinicians are working more directly on the speech of young stutterers, although not necessarily on the disfluencies. There is a tendency to focus less on the parents as the focus on the child increases. Because a more balanced view prevails on the etiology of stuttering, there seems to be less blame on the parents as causative factors. The increased number of therapies for the young stutterer reflects an increase in interest in working with the child before the condition has progressed. Even though the child may spontaneously remit, clinicians want to reach stutterers early in the belief that successful therapy is more assured in the early years. Many clinicians prefer the highly organized behavior modification programs. Our impression is that such programs offer some security to clinicians who have had little guidance in treating childhood stuttering. Adams's work (1980) offers examples of ways in which a program can be worked into the clinician's own point of view when Adams combines the GILCU approach (Ryan and Van Kirk, 1978) with attention to symptoms that reflect discoordination of the speech production mechanism.

In presenting the summaries of what are, in some cases, extensive original presentations of therapy rationales and procedures, we have tried to select the salient points and to remain objective. Our own preferences for therapy are stated in the next chapter.

ADDITIONAL THERAPY SOURCES

Space limitations have precluded the inclusion of all therapies for children. However, we recommend the following additional sources:

Conture, E. G. 1982. Stuttering. Prentice-Hall, Englewood Cliffs, N.J.

Guitar, B., and Peters, T. 1980. Stuttering: An Integration of Contemporary Therapies. Speech Foundation of America, Memphis.

Gregory, H. H., and Hill, D. 1980. Stuttering Therapy for Children. In: W. Perkins (ed.), Strategies in Stuttering Therapy. Seminars in Speech, Language and Hearing, Vol. 1, pp. 351–363. Thieme-Stratton, New York.

Luper, H. L. (ed.). 1982. Intervention with the young stutterer. J. Child. Commun. Disord. Vol. VI, no. 1.

Nelson, L. A. 1982. Evaluation of disfluency, prevention of stuttering, and management of fluency disorders in children. Paper presented at a conference sponsored by the Speech Foundation of America, Chicago.

Perkins, W. (ed.). 1980. Strategies in Stuttering Therapy. Seminars in Speech, Language and Hearing. Vol. 4. Thiemes-Stratton, New York.

Prins, D., and Ingham, R. (eds.). 1983. Treatment of Stuttering in Early Childhood: Methods and Issues. College-Hill Press: San Diego.

Starkweather, C. W. Talking with parents of young stutterers. In: J. Fraser-Gruss (ed.), Counselling Stutterers. Speech Foundation of America, Memphis.

Zwitman, D. 1978. The Disfluent Child. University Park Press, Baltimore.

REFERENCES

Adams, M. R. 1980. The young stutterer: Diagnosis, treatment and assessment of progress. Semin. Speech Lang. Hear. 1:289–300.

Andrews, G., and Harris, M. 1964. The Syndrome of Stuttering. Clinics in Developmental Medicine, no. 17, Spastics Society Medical Education and Information Unit in association with William Heineman Medical Books, London.

Andrews, G., Craig, A., Feyer, A.-M., Hoddinott, S., Howie, P., and Neilson, M. 1983. Stuttering: A review of research findings circa 1982. J. Speech Hear. Disord. 48:226–246.

Andronico, M., and Blake, I. 1971. The application of filial therapy to young children with stuttering problems. J. Speech Hear. Disord. 36:377–381.

Bloodstein, O. 1960a. The development of stuttering: I. Changes in nine basic features. J. Speech Hear. Disord. 25:219–237.

Bloodstein, O. 1960b. The development of stuttering. II: Developmental phases. J. Speech Hear. Disord. 25:366–376.

Bloodstein, O. 1961. The development of stuttering. III. Theoretical and clinical implications. J. Speech Hear. Disord. 26:67–82.

Bloodstein, O. 1981. A Handbook on Stuttering. 3rd Ed. National Easter Seal Society, Chicago.

Bluemel, C. S. 1932. Primary and Secondary Stammering. Q. J. Speech. 18:187–200.

Bluemel, C. S. 1957. The Riddle of Stuttering. Interstate Publishing Company, Danville, Ill.

Brown, S. F. 1945. The loci of stutterings in the speech sequence. J. Speech Disord. 10:181–191.

Cooper, E. B. 1965. Structured therapy for therapist and stuttering child. J. Speech Hear. Disord. 30:75–78.

Cooper, E. B. 1979. Intervention procedures for the young stutterer. In H. H. Gregory (ed.), Controversies About Stuttering Therapy, pp. 63–96. University Park Press, Baltimore.

Dell, C. W. 1980. Treating the School Age Stutterer: A Guide for Clinicians. Speech Foundation of America, Memphis.

Eisenson, J., and Horowitz, E. 1945. The influence of propositionality on stuttering. J. Speech Disord. 10:193–197.

Frick, J. V. 1970. Motor Planning Techniques for the Treatment of Stuttering. Manuscript, Pennsylvania State University.

Guerney, B. 1964. Filial therapy: Description and rationale. J. Consult. Psychol. 28:303–310.

Guitar, B., and Peters, T. J. 1980. Stuttering: An Integration of Contemporary Therapies. Speech Foundation of America, Memphis.

Johnson, L. J. 1980. Facilitating parental involvement in the therapy of the disfluent child. Semin. Speech Lang. Hear. 1:301–309.

Johnson, W. 1946. People in Quandaries. Harper & Row, New York.

Johnson, W. 1949. An open letter to the mother of a stuttering child. J. Speech Disord. 14:3–8.

Johnson, W. 1955. Stuttering in Children and Adults. University of Minnesota Press, Minneapolis.

Johnson, W. and Associates. 1959. The Onset of Stuttering. University of Minnesota Press, Minneapolis.

Johnson, W. 1967. Stuttering. In: W. Johnson and D. Moeller (eds.), Speech Handicapped School Children, 3rd Ed, pp. 229–239. Harper & Row, New York.

Kidd, K. K. 1980. Genetic models of stuttering. J. Fluency Disord. 5:187–202.

Luper, M. L., and Mulder, R. L. 1964. Stuttering: Therapy for Children. Prentice-Hall, Englewood Cliffs, N.J.

Mowrer, D. E. 1979. A Program to Establish Fluent Speech. Charles E. Merrill Publishers, Columbus, Ohio.

Ryan. B. P. 1971. Operant procedures applied to stuttering therapy for children. J. Speech Hear. Disord. 36:264–280.

Ryan, B. P. 1979. Stuttering therapy in a framework of operant conditioning and programmed learning. In: H. H. Gregory (ed.), Controversies About Stuttering Therapy, pp. 129–174. University Park Press, Baltimore.

Ryan, B., and Van Kirk, B. 1974. The establishment, transfer, and maintenance of fluent speech in 50 stutterers using delayed auditory feedback and operant procedures. J. Speech Hear. Disord. 39:3–10.

Ryan, B., and Van Kirk, B. 1978. Monterey Fluency Program. Monterey Learning Systems, Palo Alto, Calif.

Shine, R. E. 1980. Direct management of the beginning stutterer. Semin. Speech Lang. Hear. 1:339–350.

Stocker, B. 1980. The Stocker Probe Technique: For Diagnosis and Treatment of Stuttering in Young Children. Modern Education Corporation, Tulsa.

Van Riper, C. 1963. Speech Correction: Principles and Methods. 4th Ed. Prentice-Hall, Englewood Cliffs, N.J.

Van Riper, C. 1973. The Treatment of Stuttering. Prentice-Hall, Englewood Cliffs, N.J.

Webster, R. L. 1979. Empirical considerations regarding stuttering therapy. In: H. H. Gregory (ed.), Controversies About Stuttering Therapy, pp. 209–239. University Park Press, Baltimore.

Williams, D. E. 1957. A point of view about stuttering. J. Speech Hear. Disord. 22:390–397.

Williams, D. 1971. Stuttering therapy for children. In: L. E. Travis (ed.), Handbook of Speech Pathology and Audiology, pp. 1073–1096. Appleton-Century-Crofts, New York.

Williams, D. 1979. A perspective on approaches to stuttering therapy. In: H. H. Gregory (ed.), Controversies About Stuttering Therapy, pp. 241–268. University Park Press, Baltimore.

Wingate, M. E. 1976. Stuttering: Theory and Treatment. Irvington Publishers, New York.

8
Therapy for the Child Stutterer

THE CLINICIAN'S CHOICES

After the speech of the preschool child has been evaluated, clinicians have several options. If the child's speech, language, and fluency are assessed as being within normal limits, the parents may be counseled to that effect, the clinician clarifying points about acquisition in those areas and dealing with other concerns. This may be accomplished in one session, but more may be indicated. Even in such benign cases as this first example, a followup visit or at least a telephone followup is advisable in about 2 months, to check on the parents' concern and to ascertain their current view of the child's fluency.

Now assume that the preschooler's fluency pattern falls into that gray area between normal nonfluency and pathological disfluency, and a definitive diagnosis of stuttering cannot be made. The parents seem to be responsive, caring individuals, and the environment stable. In this case also, we would be inclined to counsel the parents and to see the child and parents again about 2 months hence. Following reevaluation of the child and any audiotapes made of his or her spontaneous speech by the parents, a decision regarding therapy would be made. Factors that influence us in accepting the "gray area" child for therapy include: the presence of a language-speech delay; the presence of numerous fluency disrupters in the environment, such as talkative, unsympathetic siblings; a known family history of stuttering; and the persistence of questionable disfluencies or deterioration of the condition over a period of 2 to 3 months. If we think the child is even mildly at risk, we intervene therapeutically without delay, since the child's symptoms and parental anxiety may escalate quickly.

In counseling the parents of a potential stutterer we cover areas mentioned in Chapter 6. The areas include, for example, speech, language, and fluency acquisition; situations that tend to disrupt the child's fluency; parental and child reactions to stuttering; and the influence of parental language and speech use on the child's fluency. Such topics are covered fully later in this chapter. In addition, conventional methods of reinforcing fluency are suggested. These include giving the child pleasant talking experiences on his fluent days; and providing relaxed, easy "talk-times" at an appropriate time of the day, perhaps before going to bed, when stories can be read and picture books discussed.

If the preschooler is diagnosed as a stutterer and is accepted for therapy, twice weekly sessions of one-half to one hour are scheduled for the child. Our preference is 2 hours per week. With a very young child, say a 3-year-old, we begin with 2 half-hours and work up to 2 full hours when appropriate. Individual counseling sessions are scheduled weekly for the parents for approximately 6 weeks, with the sessions tapering off to every other week at about that time. The frequency of sessions, however, varies according to need. Counseling is carried out by a speech-language pathologist, with referral to other appropriate professional services if there is a chronic disorder with the child or in the family.

Usually the diagnosis of stuttering in the school-aged child is a simpler matter than in the preschool child, and the choices of how to proceed are fewer. Questions seem to arise, however, about the very mild stutterer, and sometimes about the child who begins to stutter later, perhaps at 8 or 9 years, than at the most usual time of 3 to 5 years. In the case of the mild stutterer, the clinician may feel that there is little to offer, that the child is speaking as well as many of those who have been discharged from therapy. Because reactions to stuttering may be severe, and because of the chance that acquired behaviors will complicate the symptoms, we recommend including even the mildest stutterer in the caseload. The child who begins to stutter at the age of 8 years or so may develop symptoms rapidly. (This is based on observation; we know of no supportive research.) Because these children may build up severe secondary symptoms within a year of apparent onset, we suggest that they be accepted for therapy, or if this is deemed unsuitable by the clinician, that they be monitored closely on a followup basis.

OVERVIEW OF THERAPY

Our therapy is eclectic, but it has a language-based orientation for both preschool and school-aged children. This approach is used regardless of whether a language disorder accompanies the stuttering. However, the approach is modified if the child has a language delay. We use a combination of fluency-enhancing techniques and techniques to modify the blocking, depending on the need, as do Gregory and Hill (1980) and Guitar and Peters (1980). The fluency-enhancing techniques dovetail well with the language-based approach, and we believe that modification techniques are necessary because the stutterer is not always able to prevent blocks from occurring and needs tools to handle such situations. This applies particularly to the older child and to the more severe stutterer. When the client has even modest control over speech production, generalization activities are introduced to help reinforce the newer speech skills in life situations. After discharge, followup appointments continue for up to 2 years.

Our sessions with young stutterers are low structured; we introduce a higher structure later if we think it would be beneficial to the child, as, for example, with a young child who develops a more task-oriented attitude to therapy. Base rates of stuttering are taken at the onset of therapy and periodically during therapy. They are, however, regarded as only one dimension of progress (another being, e.g., adjustment to speaking situations at home) and are viewed within the limitations of the situations where they were acquired. That is, the base rate of stuttering recorded in the clinical setting may be different from that recorded when the child is in conversation at home. Although the clinician, and sometimes the child, may count blocks during the session, this is not done at the expense of the clinician's interaction with the child. Sessions are audiotaped for later review, and sometimes videotaped.

Clinicians select their own method of reinforcement. Usually verbal reinforcement is used, such as "I like that," "I like the way you said that," or "That was nice and easy." Reinforcement while learning a new task is consistent (100%) and then variable, to strengthen the learning.

More specific details of therapy, which includes parental counseling, are outlined according to the three factors previously discussed, namely, the psychosocial, physiological, and psycholinguistic factors. It is emphasized that all three factors will not be useful for all clients. Techniques that "fit" the client's evaluation profile should be selected as deemed appropriate by the clinician.

THE PSYCHOSOCIAL FACTOR

Who Might Be Counseled?

It is important that all significant people involved with a young stutterer be incorporated into counseling, because of the possibility that some environmental interactions may serve to maintain or exacerbate the stuttering. Usually the mother of the child is the person most available. However, many fathers of young stutterers spontaneously rearrange their schedules to participate in diagnostic counseling sessions. In addition to the immediate family, relatives who visit frequently may have an impact on the child and his communication. Relatives may be critical and nagging or loving and concerned. Either way it is imperative that they become informed, and it is best if this occurs firsthand with the clinician. The alternative is to help the parents to deal with the situation so that the child is spared well-intended, but possibly painful, attention to speech.

The significant impact of child-parental interaction is exemplified by a 7-year-old severe female stutterer, whose mother insisted over a period of months that the father's schedule did not permit him to attend counseling sessions. Finally, when we were becoming extremely disgruntled and concerned about the child's lack of progress, we insisted on a joint conference. The father was a likable but tired and tense gentleman, who could not tolerate listening to or watching stuttering. He had approved, admired, and encouraged any tricks or devices that his daughter used to get even fleeting fluency. It was clear that none of our counseling with the mother had filtered through to her husband, and she had described his reactions to the stuttering as "slightly impatient at times." After lengthy discussion, the father realized that he was unwittingly sabotaging therapy with the girl, who had developed such an elaborate array of antiexpectancy devices to prevent stuttering from occurring, that she was difficult to communicate with, quite apart from her stuttering.

The information that the parents bring to the counseling sessions, and their thoughts on their child's communication difficulties, are essential to the effectiveness of the sessions. However, we do have information that they need, and we impart it as clearly as possible. Following the format of the evaluation chapter, areas are outlined containing examples of questions and problems that may arise in such sessions. We include some of our responses and ways of dealing with the children on specific issues.

Dealing with the Child's "Knowledge" of Stuttering

It is difficult to generalize, but many of the preschool stutterers we accept into therapy indicate in some way that they are aware of stuttering. We can offer some examples. The mother of one 3-year-old child described severe, nonvocal blocks, when his mouth was fixed in an open position while he tried to force the sound through. Although the blocking was present each day, it occurred relatively infrequently, and the mother did not think that the boy was aware of it. The child was reasonably fluent on the first visit, and we saw him several times for evaluation. During the third informal play session, he exhibited the symptom in addition to several milder disfluencies. The block was very forceful, and it certainly seemed likely that he felt it. After he had forced the word out, he glanced surreptitiously at the clinician to see if she had also noticed. When she commented that "It really looked hard to say that," the child set down his toy, looked at her with relief and said, "Yes, it was. That happens to me sometimes and I don't know why it does, do you?"

Not all children will be as open as this boy when reference is made to speech breakdowns. One 4-year-old responded to a similar overture with "I think I gotta go now." This reaction obviously reflected the child's sensitivity to the stuttering, and we were able to pace the directness of our therapy with him accordingly. The clinician clearly needs to be intuitive about whether to refer directly to hard speech and when to do so. However, when there are overt signs of awareness it seems insensitive *not* to acknowledge the stuttering. Children may be relieved by the openness and are unlikely to be hurt by it.

It is difficult to know what the young stutterer feels about stuttering. We think that he or she may feel concern, perhaps verging on fear, and at times frustration. Unlike the older stutterer who is aware of, and can think about, the concept of stuttering, the youngster deals with a more rudimentary idea of "My words are stuck in my throat, can you see them?" In addition to a possibly direct approach with the child, the clinician might also relieve concern about speech indirectly, by working with the parents on *their* reactions to the stuttering. In the foregoing example of the girl who developed an array of antiexpectancy devices, therapy gains were made when we secured her father's understanding of the difficulty and support for what we were all trying to accomplish. Most important, helping to increase fluency and the control of speech will improve the child's self-image as a speaker.

The school-aged child usually "knows," of course, that he or she stutters. The extent to which the condition is likely to be acknowledged probably depends on a number of factors. Some 10- or 12-year-olds surprise clinicians with their observations about stuttering and their acute self-appraisal. Others tend to look around the room at the mention of "stuttering," as though searching for some other person to whom this description applies—*they* are certainly just part of the group and have no unusual or outstanding characteristics drawing attention to themselves. It is possible for this apparent lack of involvement in the topic of stuttering to be viewed as a lack of motivation. Clinicians should be cautious, however, about using "lack of motivation" as a reason for not doing therapy, or for accounting for therapy failure. Too often this becomes a wastebasket term to excuse our failures with stutterers.

Dealing with the Child's Reactions to Stuttering

Although some situations, on the whole, seem to disrupt young stutterers' speech more than others, the level of awareness of situational influences in the preschool child probably is fairly low. At least we have no evidence of either speech (sound, word cues), or situational awareness, occasional observations of word substitution or circumlocution notwithstanding. Two of the known consistent disrupters of fluency in these youngsters are excitement and fatigue. We deal now with the larger, global disrupters that clearly influence the control of speech production, and move on to the more subtle pragmatic influences in the psycholinguistic factor section.

When parents become aware of the association between excitement and increased disfluency they can usually modify disrupting influences in the household. This seems to be advisable until the child has stabilized fluency. It is usually a good idea to reduce, for example, play periods of very high excitement. We had one 3-year-old in therapy who was very small for his age. We wondered how he survived the nightly romps with his athletic father, who described throwing the child high in the air and catching him, and other physical gymnastics that could verge on violence. The play sometimes reached a frenzied level, and the child's speech markedly deteriorated. After discussion, the father decided to reduce this rough-house play to avoid instigating the child's stuttering. Similarly, most parents are willing to make schedule adjustments for themselves and for the child to allow the child to get adequate sleep, if fluency seems to be affected by fatigue.

As previously stated, school-aged stutterers usually know that they stutter, but they are thought to have less awareness of the details of stuttering than adult stutterers. They are also less able to predict its occurrence in conversation (Bloodstein, 1981) and in reading (Silverman and Williams, 1972). Van Riper's tracks and Bloodstein's phases suggest that avoidances accrue over time as the child matures. Certainly with the teenager, and even with the younger stutterer, one must be prepared to encounter avoidances. Even 10-year-old stutterers have been known to possess sophisticated and subtle devices designed to "interiorize" the stuttering (Douglass and Quarrington, 1952).

We begin work on avoidances of words, sounds, and situations, if present, as soon as the child demonstrates some increase in fluency and control over the blocks. Desensitization to situations is arranged hierarchically as suggested by Van Riper (1973), with the easiest situations first and then the more difficult situations. Before asking our young clients to enter a feared situation outside the clinic, we role play the situation. For example, Sue needs to get up and read orally in front of the class, using loose contacts. She does it first with her clinician, simulating the classroom atmosphere as much as possible. Next, the audience size is gradually increased so that the situation is more realistic. And finally she tries out her oral reading at school in the classroom. If appropriate, and with her consent, we alert the teacher to the fact that Sue is ready to try something new, or in a different way, so that the teacher can facilitate matters if necessary.

Sometimes we can take advantage of situations that arise that were not part of the original hierarchical plan. One 15-year-old male auditioned for a school play and got precisely the part he wanted. He was then afraid that he would not be able to handle it. For several weeks he practiced his part with his clinician, who filled in all the other parts, while the client aimed at using loose contacts and easy coarticulatory movements. This was a more meaningful and effective therapy step for him than the original step in the hierarchical plan would have been.

Teaching children to react constructively to disfluencies in various situations rather than with the "old" reactions of apprehension or fear constitutes a large part of the generalization of therapy. The extent and kinds of reaction, however, seem to be related to age and to the severity of the symptoms, and perhaps to factors that are less easy to describe and talk about, such as personality type.

Dealing with Parental Reactions to Stuttering

Parents' reactions to their children's stuttering can run the gamut of embarrassment, shame, fear, and guilt, or simply appropriate concern. Many parents come in with the question "Did I (we) cause the stuttering?" Sometimes they have read material that espoused a particular viewpoint—usually that stutterers are the product of their environment. Sometimes they have talked to friends or other professionals who have presented that view. We try to find out the kind of information they have, where it came from, and what they think they might have done to "cause" the stuttering. Some perspective on the topic usually emerges from such discussions. Frequently the parents need information on the possible etiologies of stuttering and reassurance that in spite of our being unable to identify a specific "cause," the condition is amenable to treatment.

Occasionally we find a parent with whom this kind of discussion is not fruitful. An example of this was a divorced mother who insisted that her 4-year-old son's stuttering was caused by her former husband's behavior when living in the home, and the subsequent arguments and separation. Regardless of whether this was "the cause," it became clear as the session progressed that the mother's anger at her former husband was preventing productive discussion about the child's difficulties. During the first weeks of therapy this was observed as a consistent pattern, and additionally, other family problems emerged. We referred the family to a resource appropriate for the wide range of adjustment problems presented, and continued the child in therapy for stuttering and related disorders.

One of the most frequent reactions of parents to their child's stuttering is a difficulty in dealing with the topic with the child. Such parents might say "I don't know what to do when he stutters. Should I say anything? And if so, what?" Usually the parents would like to respond in some way to the child's distress, but perhaps because of lack of information, or because they have been warned that the stuttering must be ignored, they stay silent and somewhat distressed themselves. This can occur with a disfluent child of any age. Once again we explore what the parents have been doing and ask about the advice they have been given. Sometimes they have found their own way and have begun to make comments such as "I'll listen, so take your time." If parents are responding like this in a nonpunitive way, with no ill effect on the child, we leave the situation as it is. If the parents are directing possible negative attention to the stuttering or introducing punitive measures, we ask them to desist until we know the child a little better and can work out with them the most constructive ways for them to help. As parents observe therapy, they note (or are shown) that the clinician occasionally comments "That looked a bit hard to say" and perhaps suggests that the child use "easy speech." With an older child who may be in distress because of stuttering, the parental comment might be "You certainly seem to be having a rough time with your speech today." This help, however, is timed to coincide with what the clinician is doing in therapy, and the results of the parents' intervention are discussed with them, so that adaptations can be made if necessary. The parents are now openly acknowledging the stuttering, and the child probably is relieved that the growing tension has been reduced. Frequently the parents' sympathetic comment, in addition to easing the tension, is a tacit reminder to the child to monitor the speech pattern and to put into practice techniques that have been taught in therapy. As therapy progresses, the parents are provided with more information and observation of therapy sessions so that they can be attuned to what the child can do, and further ways that they might help.

Parents may also report feeling impatient at times with their child's stuttering, particularly when they are extremely busy and the youngster wants to begin a long discussion. Under these circumstances, most parents apparently feel obliged to stop their activity and attend to the child. We suggest that the child be told, in a reassuring way, that this is not a good time to talk and that the parent will be glad to discuss the topic a little later. Once parents have been introduced to this casual and practical way of dealing with such dilemmas (one that has been well described by Ginott, 1965) life frequently becomes simpler, and no harm is done to the child.

A further pertinent observation of parental reactions was made by L. A. Nelson at a conference sponsored by the Speech Foundation of America (1982). She noted that when interacting with the child, parents and also clinicians must omit from their vocabularies words that reflect value judgments. That is, rather than using words such as "good," "bad," "right," "wrong," or "nice," to describe the child's behavior, praise him or her for the interesting things accomplished, such as drawings, or ideas that the child has shared.

Dealing with Parental Language and Speech Use

If parents are fast talkers, they are asked to slow down their rate of speech. If their conversation is highly sophisticated, and they habitually talk beyond the semantic-syntactic level of the child, they are requested to simplify their conversation. With a second clinician, they observe therapy through a one-way screen or on closed-circuit video and discuss the ways in which the clinician doing therapy adapts her speaking rate and language use to facilitate fluency in the child.

Other methods of facilitating fluency are discussed. For example, an open-ended question such as "Why are you putting your trucks into that box instead of the other one?" requires a complex response. That question is more likely to elicit stuttering than an either/or question, requiring a one-word phrase or response, or a yes/no question. The parents' strategically placed comments or easy questions may also help the child to gain some control over his speech when relating a long story. Many parents feel particularly helpless at this time, not wanting to interrupt the story, yet observing increasing discomfort and disfluency as the child moves into more complex material. An occasional comment or simple question about the content of the story may be enough to have the child pause, and allow the excitement of the story to subside.

The Child's Interactions with Others

Some possible interactions of the child with parents and relatives have been discussed. Relationships with peers, siblings, and teachers may or may not be limited by the stuttering. Our experience is that it takes an extremely secure young school-aged stutterer not to be affected in some way by peer teasing. The child may have basically good relationships with peers, but may need help in coping with this area to maintain or reestablish satisfactory interactions.

Preschoolers are less likely to be teased (unless they have an extremely severe communication disorder or older playmates) because teasers tend to be school-aged children from 6 or 7 years on. Most of the therapeutic thrust at handling teasing is therefore directed at the schoolchild. This should be regarded as an important area of therapy because its impact can be strong on individual children. For example, a 7-year-old female stutterer seemed to be developing a school phobia when we first met her. It centered around her wish to avoid a particular group of boys in her class who teased her about her speech from the moment she arrived at school. She was reluctant to attend school and insisted that her mother drive her there, timing her arrival precisely to coincide with the moment the other children had entered the class.

We deal with teasing through direct discussion with the child and through the child role playing with the clinician. The clinician and the child take turns at playing the teaser and the teased. In this way the clinician can demonstrate alternate ways for the child to respond to taunts and give the child clues about the motives of the teaser. A 6- or 7-year-old can comprehend that the teaser gets a thrill and feels important on seeing somebody else squirm. He or she can also understand that if you deprive the teaser of a reaction, that power is reduced. One 8-year-old child in our care was constantly teased by an older and larger brother about his speech, among other things. Through role playing our client lost some of his fear of the situation, and began to respond to his brother by looking him squarely in the eye and saying "Is this how you get your kicks?" The teasing was reduced considerably. We try to get the child to a point of being able to respond calmly to a teaser with something like "Yes, I know I stutter. It's something I'm working on." Some children find their own way, as did a large 14-year-old who was a skilled wrestler. He commented, "No one says anything about my speech. They'd better not!"

Many children have been told to "ignore" teasing. We think this is virtually impossible. The child cannot ignore the teasing any more than the parent can ignore the stuttering. The school-aged stutterers may be desensitized to it, as described above, and given alternate responses to use, and ample help and support. In this way they will not feel so trapped when they see the bully approaching. Eventually, this situation should be a challenge during the generalization stage of therapy!

Parents report that sibling relationships can be strained intermittently by specific situations. For the stutterer, one of the situations of strain is usually that of verbal competition with fluent brothers and sisters. The most intense competition usually takes place at the dinner table. The simple introduction of turn-taking, imposed and enforced by the parents, may resolve the problem. Ultimately, as with the teasing, this would be an ideal generalization situation for young stutterers—that is, to insist on their turn and to control the speech pattern. Initially, and certainly for the young stutterer, parental intervention is necessary.

Simple solutions are, of course, not always readily available for problems of interaction with significant people in one's environment, and, in some cases, special help is required. On the other hand, not all the situations described here exist with all stutterers.

The Child's Overall Adjustment

The clinician should endeavor to keep an open mind in this area. The assumption, for instance, that young stutterers have perfectionistic parents has been a popular and sometimes justified point of view. However, this characteristic has not been substantiated in the majority of parents studied (see Chapter 1). Most stutterers are fairly normal youngsters who happen to have a hard time talking. However, because we must be aware of anything that might maintain the stuttering or worsen it, the way in which the child fits into his world is important to us. The older child may have school difficulties that directly relate to stuttering. These might include reluctance to participate orally in class and reluctance to participate socially. If these difficulties are attributable to stuttering, they should be alleviated partly as therapy progresses and fluency increases. Occasionally a child may have adjustment problems that are extreme, and perhaps unrelated to the speech disorder. For such a child, that is, one with chronic antisocial or maladaptive behavior, referral to a source skilled in handling such problems is necessary. Sometimes, as in a case cited earlier, we refer the entire family for assistance. By and large, however, we think that the speech-language pathologist can deal with the stutterer and the family.

Clinicians are sometimes concerned that parents will reject recommendations to other resources. Usually the reaction of the parents to this kind of proposal can be anticipated fairly early in therapy. We do not make such a recommendation immediately unless the parents seek it. We find that the recommendation is almost always accepted if the parents are given some time while the child is in therapy to become accustomed to us, and to evaluate the information that they receive at the clinic.

As previously stated, we believe that speech-language pathologists can handle most of the issues under the "psychosocial" heading. If a chronic adjustment problem exists, the clinician's broad background should ensure that it is recognized and an appropriate referral made. It is worthwhile to cultivate reliable sources for referral, so that your clients can get competent, professional service.

In our counseling sessions we treat the parents as co-workers on a case. Each party has information to exchange and to work with. We encourage the parents to keep us informed of any event in the child's life that may affect the therapy session, or, better still, to have the child communicate the event to the clinician if he or she is able to do so. Finally, we have the parents of young stutterers read the book *If Your Child Stutters: A Guide for Parents* (Ainsworth, 1977). It contains comprehensive information and commonsense advice.

Summary

This section has addressed direct and indirect methods of handling child, parental, and environmental reactions to stuttering. *Direct methods* include appropriate explanation to the younger child about the concept of "hard speech," increasing the child's fluency and control of stuttering, reducing situational avoidances, and dealing with teasing of the school-aged child. *Indirect methods* include information sharing with parents, reducing fluency disrupters in the environment, helping parents to talk with their children about stuttering, helping parents to deal with tense moments of stuttering, slowing down parental speech rate and reducing sentence complexity when appropriate, increasing linguistic knowledge so that they can facilitate fluency, and using bibliotherapy.

Not all material covered in this section applies to all children who stutter. The clinician's discretion is imperative in deciding which areas require intervention.

THE PHYSIOLOGICAL FACTOR

The Preschooler versus the School-aged Child

Physiological aspects of stuttering appear to be less complex in the preschool stutterer than in the older child, in that the struggle, tension, facial contortions, and severe blockings associated with many advanced stutterers have not developed. However, some researchers have defined a subgroup of young stutterers as having a motor component to the disfluencies that influences the coordination of the speech production mechanism, suggesting a need to assist the motorically involved child with speech attempts (Adams, 1980; L. A. Nelson, 1982; Riley and Riley, 1979, 1980). A simpler pattern of stuttering will exist in most young stutterers, but we have known a 3-year-old to exhibit silent, forced blocks, vocal fry, pitch breaks, tongue protrusion, eye closure, and facial contortions. Fortunately such severity is rare in one so young, and it is possible to help the "average" preschool child with the physiological components of speech production by teaching "easy speech" in the context of a slow-normal rate of speech, and a psycholinguistic framework that controls the language stimuli used. The slower rate of speech is thought to give the child more time to make the complex physiological adjustments required to synchronize the movements of the vocal tract, and in time a more variable speech rate may be introduced to therapy.

Examples of techniques for improving the respiratory, phonatory, coarticulatory, and aerodynamic factors of speech production are discussed next. The clinician must adapt the categories and techniques according to their relevance to the child and the symptoms.

Techniques for Improving Respiratory Control

Respiratory abnormalities are usually considered to be secondary to the stuttering, rendering specific work on breathing patterns unnecessary in many cases, because if the pattern is disrupted, it may normalize when the blocking is reduced. Caution is warranted in using breathing exercises with the very young child. The preschooler probably has not yet developed the adult pattern of about seven breaths per minute for conversational speech, and in general may not be expected to have precise coordination over this mechanism, like the older child or adult.

A young child may, however, force words out while using the limits of the expiratory reserve volume. An indirect way of assisting the child is to slow down the speech rate, prevent the rush of words, and encourage appropriate pauses in an utterance. Sometimes all it takes is a hand on the arm to suggest "Pause for a second." Also, by the clinician's modeling of brief linguistic units and encouraging the same from the child, "chunking" of speech—grouping words into phrases and clauses—can be encouraged, which automatically results in appropriate pauses for inhalation purposes. This begins with isolated, small chunks of speech during play, and eventually leads to story telling and conversation that incorporate appropriate pauses for respiration, so that the chances of the child's running out of breath are reduced. The appropriate sequencing of linguistic units for this respiratory work are part of the "psycholinguistic factor."

Keep in mind that the clause boundary is a vulnerable point for the young stutterer, who is more likely to incur stuttering at that point than at other points in the utterance. Helping the child to time the respiration points appropriately with the onset of clauses may help the ease with which he handles the early part of the clause. Most of this work can be done, however, indirectly.

With the older child, breathing exercises should be instituted only if the clinician detects an aberrant pattern. Clavicular breathing, for example, creating tension in the upper chest and laryngeal area, can be altered to a thoracic-abdominal pattern that will offer better support for speech production. We rarely find this change necessary, but if it is, a simple explanation of what is required is in order. It must be conveyed that the change will give the child more breath to talk with, and that the shift in focus of breathing (from the clavicular area) may reduce tension in the upper chest and neck. The child can then stand with a relaxed stance, but good posture, hand placed gently on the abdomen to feel its rise and fall with inhalation and exhalation. Feeling the out-and-in pattern of the clinician's lower thoracic or abdominal area may assist the child, if the child cannot make the change easily. If the child still experiences difficulty, lying supine and repeating the exercise usually facilitates the shift. Eventually the child must be upright, incorporating short phrases and then short sentences into the new breathing pattern.

If the school-aged child has poor timing of the respiratory cycle for speech, direct help may be required to synchronize respiration with the constituents of the sentence, that is, with the clauses and phrases. Again, a simple and direct explanation is in order. Some children are helped by reading a passage that has been marked off in clause units, which indicate where the pauses and the inhalations for speech should come. Once they have the idea, the new pattern can be reinforced in short segments of spontaneous speech, and finally in conversational speech.

Although we tend to use such direct methods with the school-aged child, L. A. Nelson (1982), working with very young children, states:

> *It may be difficult for the child to control the breath stream. I am interested in trying to devise games in which he can experience*

relaxed breathing and a return to normal breathing patterns. To begin with, we will need to try an activity that doesn't require talking. If he consents, the parent, the child, and the clinician will lie on their backs on the floor—just relaxing, certainly not "resting for sleep." We will look at the ceiling and just breathe in and out easily—no forcing, no altering of the normal pattern. When we are relaxed we can exhale the air gently—just the tiniest amount, by turn. It is important to model for a child when explanations can be unclear or not needed. The clinician can take a turn, then the parent, then the child. Then we can take turns at being a "little wind" and made the "ooooooo" sound. If the child is willing, the clinician can say a number or a word, then the child, with one exhaled breath at the start. We can aim for phrases and short sentences later

(L. A. Nelson, Speech Foundation of America Conference, 1982, p. 17).

Techniques for Improving Phonatory Control

For the young child, the concept of "easy speech" (Williams, 1971, 1979) is applied not only to the easing of tension in the upper articulators, but to the larynx also. The 4-year-old is not about to differentiate between "speech" and "phonation." The use of easy speech by the clinician—speech of slightly slowed rate, with loose articulators, gentle voice initiation, and slightly lower volume—will provide a good model for the child's phonation, which eventually should be without strain and harshness, and with easy voice initiation.

Phonation does not occur in a vacuum, and any work that is done on respiration may have both decreased vocal strain by supplying stronger breath support and released tension by slowing down the speech rate. Direct attention to coordination of the breath stream and vocal fold activity may, however, be necessary. With young children, we try to establish a reciprocal relationship so that they can have us imitate what they do, and we can have them imitate what we do. What we want them to imitate at this point is a slow, easy sigh, something like a heavily aspirated "AH." After trying this a few times, slowly and easily, we have them add voice, following our model, so that a breathy, but voiced "AH" with an exceptionally easy onset is the result. We shape that to a breathy "I"—a frequently stuttered word for young children—and, maintaining a slight breathiness on the "I," elicit short phrases such as "I'm Jimmy," "I'm five," "I'm big." When this phase of the activity begins, the clinician is still providing the model; however, most youngsters can continue this activity, at least for a brief period, generating their own "I'm—" structures. We are not fussy about accepting offbeat constructions, provided they begin with "I." If a child has difficulties with this technique, clinician and child may speak in unison, with the clinician gradually fading out and the child continuing. Each child is helped to use the word "I" at the onset of increasingly long phrases and sentences, always, of course, within the confines of his or her linguistic ability. As the clinician reduces the breathiness of the modeled "I," the child usually follows suit. The result is an easy onset on the word "I," rather than the hard attack that results from a system that is poorly coordinated at the level of the glottis. The clinician may wish to pursue this technique for the word "and," another word frequently stuttered by young stutterers. We repeat that such direct techniques are used with the pre-school child only if other less direct techniques, such as slowing down the speech rate and controlled use of linguistic units, fail to be effective.

The older child will benefit from the foregoing technique, and depending on age and maturity, may also benefit from simple explanations of the process. Physiological explanations, however, must be very carefully made because a child may misinterpret even a well-organized presentation. One child of our acquaintance went home from a therapy session somewhat upset, telling his mother that he had something in his throat that squeezed up when he talked. The analogy of the vocal tract and stuttering, in which the water hose is squeezed tightly, preventing the flow of water, can be used quite effectively in therapy (Conture, 1982). However, it is advisable to check on the child's interpretation of what you have described before the end of the session.

The easy onset technique just described is sometimes consciously adopted by older children for use in conversation because it provides a tool for handling glottal constrictions that occur on words beginning with vowels.

Techniques for Facilitating Coarticulatory and Aerodynamic Control

As stated in Chapter 5, the child's repetitions of sounds and syllables (m-m-m-mommy; mo-mo-mo-mommy) and prolongations of stuttering (mmmmommy) may be viewed as poor coarticulation in that there is a temporary cessation of overlapping articulatory gestures that are normally associated with fluent speech production: "Coarticulation and adaptation of one articulatory movement to another is pervasive in running speech" (Borden and Harris, 1980, p. 128).

Although abnormally slowed speech rate, as is practiced in some rate control therapies, may create another kind of coarticulatory difficulty, our experience is that the slow-normal rate of speech—perhaps incurring a "simplification of motor timing" (Adams, 1980)—usually reduces the number of repetitions and prolongations of sounds in the young stutterer's speech. That is, coarticulation occurs more easily in these circumstances.

The technique may also contribute to the coarticulatory ease of the older or more advanced stutterer.

More specific techniques to foster coarticulatory ease include loose contacts and pullouts. Like Van Riper (1973) and Luper and Mulder (1964), we find loose contacts a most useful technique, one that can be demonstrated to children of almost any age. The technique requires reduction of muscle activity in the vocal tract, thereby preventing immobilizing tension and allowing smooth movement through the word. With the very young child we use floppy rag dolls and puppets; clinicians, assuming a relaxed, "floppy" posture, make movements to suggest muscle looseness. We show them loose contacts for speech production and ask them to try it—to talk as though they are very tired. Having the child talk "easy" instead of "hard" is another way of getting at loose contacts.

The older, more severe stutterer may imagine that the lips are not even going to touch. For example, for the initial "b" sound of "bye," the child would aim to produce the word by almost (but not quite) closing the lips. If there is habitually much overshoot in the lip muscle for this sound, the lips will approximate anyway, but more lightly than usual. The lightness of the contact prevents fixation or tremor and allows appropriate coarticulatory movement to occur. When the loose contacts have been reinforced in the customary manner, with increasing length and complexity of the linguistic units, the child will practice them in conversation. Even the very young child can learn to reduce the tension of speaking at a sign from the clinician to "stay loose." Parents of preschoolers, as well as their clinicians, have observed these youngsters beginning to tense up for talking, and then spontaneously—without external help—loosen themselves before speech.

As a backup to loose contacts for fostering articulatory movement through the word, Van Riper's pullout is particularly useful for the school-aged stutterer. Recall that Van Riper specified that childhood stutterers may be taught "how to ease out of their repetitions or blockages slowly and smoothly" (Van Riper, 1973, p. 444). Sometimes clinicians are bothered by pullouts if the child is not immediately proficient with them. Because the pullout is such a useful technique, we suggest that the clinician simply find another way to teach it. First, a simple explanation is required. For example:

> *Pushing your way out of a block doesn't really help. It's a habit and it's uncomfortable. Instead of pushing, ease the word out and move gently onto the rest of the word. You need to loosen up—like a loose contact right there in the middle of the block. But don't forget to get moving and finish the rest of the word.*

If the child cannot pull out after explanation and demonstration, stutter with the child and have him or her follow you out of the block. When the client becomes proficient with the technique, it will be valuable in coping with unanticipated blocks.

Finally, we use cancellation (defined in Chapter 7) for the preschooler in an extremely modified form. The technique allows the child to reattempt a word in which the articulatory gestures have not been smoothly produced. When clients know the difference between hard and easy speech, it is a simple matter to say after a hard block, "That looked hard, try it over the easy way." If they need assistance at first in saying it over, model the easy way, or say it with them. We suggest that this is a sensible approach when children talk "hard" at home, when playing with friends, or anywhere. They are shown how to use this form of cancellation and encouraged to use it, but we do not intellectualize with the youngsters. We never nag, and never make them feel guilty about something they cannot do, or do not wish to do. If a child responds to the intervention as one 4-year-old did, with "I gotta go the bathroom NOW," the clinician may respond with "You don't want to try that now. OK, go to the bathroom. You can try your easy speech later." The same child may participate happily a little later, or even try the technique of his or her own accord.

With the older child, more formal practice with cancellation is in order. Many children resent "stuttering again," which is often their erroneous interpretation of the second part of the original cancellation, so we simply require a production in the direction of fluency. That is, the child blocks on a word in conversation or reading, stops and pauses momentarily, and then repeats the word in the direction of fluency, or perhaps fluently. When children use this technique it signifies that they are monitoring their speech—no small accomplishment—and because they have in memory the fluent or nearly fluent production, fluency rather then stuttering is being reinforced. The result seems to be a reduction in the severity and frequency of the blocks.

So now, in addition to the basic therapy paradigm of slower, easier speech on increasing linguistic units, children have three methods of dealing with the disfluencies, thanks to Van Riper. If they use loose contacts much of the time and this becomes a habit, they reduce the frequency and severity of the blocks. If, however, they get into a block, they can pull out; failing that, they can cancel. That is effective control.

Assuming that the child has adequate breath support for speech, that there is a reduction in the tension and constriction of the vocal tract, and that there are smoother coarticulatory movements for speech occurring without abnormal occlusion of the tract, the aerodynamics of speech production should normalize. Recall that vocal tract tension, constriction, and occlusion result in aberrant airflow rates and vocal tract pressures. However, when the vocal tract parts are moving smoothly and in synchrony, the airflow for speech should be automatically regulated by the vocal tract.

Techniques for Reducing Associated Symptoms

The associated characteristics of stuttering tend to straddle the three factors—psychosocial, physiological, and psycholinguistic. Situational avoidances were covered under the psychosocial factor. Some associated characteristics, however, are more physiological than others. Physical movements such as eye closure and body movement, for example, tend to subside as the child learns to approach and carry out speech production without force and tension. For children whose secondary behaviors persist, usually the older children, we follow Van Riper's example in having them learn to identify a characteristic. If they postpone production of a word by saying "ah ah ah," for instance, we have them engage in a few minutes of conversation with the clinician using an automatic counter (the kind golfers use), or a pencil and paper. Their task is to count the number of times the postponement device is used. The tally is checked with that of the clinician. If they have identified the device accurately, they move on to attempting a brief conversation with the clinician without using the device, but instead, moving onto each word with an easy onset. If conversation is too difficult, simpler activities are indicated, such as imitating sentences modeled by the clinician without using the device, or answering simple questions. Or, the client might be asked to gradually reduce the number of "ah's" inserted into an utterance (a shaping procedure), or to temporarily exaggerate the symptom. In exaggeration, instead of repeating the "ah" the usual three times, it is repeated four times, or five times (a massing procedure). Awareness of the device is considerably heightened by exaggeration, and the client may begin to recognize the symptom upon finding the mouth open for that first "ah." This response indicates that the massed practice (i.e., the voluntary, repeated production of a behavior (response) in the absence of reinforcement, to achieve extinction of that behavior) is being effective.

If the stutterer is to eradicate the secondary characteristics, however, he or she must have techniques for handling the blocks. It is unfair to ask the client to relinquish the secondaries if there is no way to cope with what is left. In our experience, working on the secondary symptoms may not be popular with children. It seems to be serious and difficult work. We therefore feel indulgent when clinicians and clients "ham it up" to lighten therapy a little. Nonaudible characteristics, such as eye blinks, may also be incorporated into the foregoing approach.

Summary

Therapy under the physiological factor stresses the use of a slow-normal rate of speech to aid more appropriate respiratory, phonatory, coarticulatory, and aerodynamic control for speech production. The concept of "easy" speech versus "hard" speech is promoted for children of all ages. For respiration, the child is taught to make appropriate pauses for speech breathing, to correct any aberrant breathing patterns, and to synchronize inhalation and exhalation with production of an utterance. For both younger and older children, the clinician teaches easy onset of phonation by shaping a sigh to a breathy vowel, to a word, and to a phrase beginning with the word. Van Riper's modification techniques of loose contacts, pullouts, and cancellations are used with the older or more severe stutterer; modified versions are suggested for the younger stutterer. Techniques for modifying the blocks may be usefully incorporated into language units of increasing length and complexity. Associated characteristics that do not subside spontaneously are dealt with through a variety of behavior modification techniques.

THE PSYCHOLINGUISTIC FACTOR

General Considerations

The association of a psycholinguistic factor and stuttering emanates from a number of events that were described in Chapter 4. In brief, the events are: observations and research on the nonfluencies of normal speech and language development, syntactic influences on the nonfluencies in the speech of fluent or highly nonfluent normally speaking children, the slower rate of speech-language acquisition in some young stutterers, and the relation of the points of speech breakdown to the constituent structure of the sentence. In addition, clinicians have noted that stutterers achieve fluency more easily on shorter units of speech than on longer and presumably more complex units. Apparently young stutterers have noticed this also; researchers have found a preponderance of one-word utterances in the spontaneous speech of these youngsters (Kline and Starkweather, 1979; Wall, 1980), although this finding might also suggest a delay in language acquisition.

The following points need to be considered when embarking on a therapy program with the young stutterer: the child may be withholding vocabulary and sentence structures in an effort to control the stuttering; there may be a speech and language lag; the child's rate of stuttering may be influenced by the length and by the semantic-syntactic complexity of the utterance; the stuttering may occur at predictable places in the utterance, primarily at clause boundaries; the child may have developed an individual pattern of stuttering related to pragmatic events.

Considerations of a Speech and Language Delay

Many young stutterers exhibit difficulties in sound production (see Blood-stein, 1981, for a review) that, if mild and not interfering with intelligibility, may be dealt with when the child's fluency has stabilized. The youngster who exhibits an intelligibility problem, however, requires intervention because lack of intelligibility may add considerable strain and effort to his communicative attempts. This applies to children who are considered to have articulation disorders as well as to those with phonological problems. Clinicians are sometimes reluctant to work on symptoms other than stuttering in the preschooler, lest attention to speech and/or language worsen the stuttering. For the most part, this fear appears to be unjustified. There are, however, reports of speech- and language-delayed children who have exhibited stuttering or stuttering-like behavior after a period of therapy.

Therapy for the multiply disordered child needs to be sensibly organized and carefully paced. For example, the sound or sound group selected for attention must be motorically the simplest and easiest for the child to produce. Similarly the stimuli (words and phrases) chosen should be on a level that the child can easily cope with. Help for the stuttering can be integrated with the work on sound production. For example, loose contacts or easy speech may be encouraged while the child tries out his new sounds and words containing the sounds. Of course it is possible to "overload" a child, stutterer or not, with complex linguistic stimuli, and that is certainly a danger.

One of the authors observed a beginning student clinician in a therapy session with a fluent child who had an articulation disorder. The student had taught the client to say the word "comb" successfully, using his new /k/ sound. She then asked him to say the sentence "I know how to comb my hair." His response was: "I comb my hair." She tried again and received the same response. Then she emphasized "I KNOW HOW to comb my hair." With visible tension the child responded with "I KNOW——comb my hair."

The novice clinician had insufficient knowledge of sequencing the steps of therapy, and instead of moving the child to a two- or three-word structure, she had swamped him with a complex sentence, not to mention a pragmatically inappropriate stimulus. The child, who was 5 years old, demonstrated perhaps a less than average capacity for recall or ability to deal with the complexity of the sentence. We refer to this kind of strain imposed on a child as "linguistic overload," for want of a better term. The child's apparent uncertainty and strain may be similar to that which occurs when language-delayed youngsters develop disfluencies during language therapy. It is emphasized that the clinician needs comprehensive knowledge of the language and sound system, how it develops, and how it may interact with therapy, to provide help for the multiply disordered youngster.

For the child who has a language delay, difficulties with semantic-syntactic structures in spontaneous speech can be expected. As the child's fluency level improves, new structures may be incorporated gradually into therapy, with the clinician monitoring the effects of language increases on the child's fluency.

Increasing Linguistic Units

Many recent therapies use the successive increase of language units as a means of facilitating fluency (Gregory and Hill, 1980; Mowrer, 1979; Ryan and Van Kirk, 1978; Shine, 1980; Stocker, 1980), and it is worthwhile to explore the ramifications of this practice. The therapy begins by having the child produce one word, the clinician being aware that the child invariably will be fluent on a solitary word. When fluency on one-word units has been satisfactorily reinforced, the utterance is extended to two words, then to three words, and so on. Note the number of variables that may change with this increase in length. The motor planning required to coordinate the respiratory, phonatory, articulatory, and coarticulatory systems becomes increasingly complex. Then, with the longer utterances, semantic-syntactic complexity usually increases. (It is possible, of course, to have a one-word utterance that is semantically complex—for example, "Courage!" And we have all listened to lengthy sentences that say very little.) Longer sentences can evolve to some extent by phrase additions using the simple conjoiner "and," but the connection of subordinate or coordinate clauses and the insertion of embedded clauses usually makes sentences longer. It is more common, therefore, to have simple sentences of modest length. With an increase in the length of the sentence we expect an increase in the motor planning required for the sentence, and an increase in the semantic-syntactic complexity of the sentence. Underlying all this, presumably, is an increase in cognitive activity. The variables involved in lengthening the sentence cannot be controlled entirely. From the point of view of the physiology of speech and the cognitive underpinnings of language, and the interaction of the two that takes place, however, it makes sense to be sensitive to the multiple issues involved in increasing the length of an utterance. The following more specific description of therapy techniques for the preschool child is based on considerations of utterance length and semantic-syntactic complexity.

First, the child and the clinician engage in play in a low structured setting. The child is encouraged to participate and to talk. If the child is uncomfortable at first with interactive play, parallel play is used. During the session the clinician's speech is slow-normal—not abnormally slow—

to provide an appropriate model for the child. The clinician then finds ways to elicit short one- or two-word utterances from the child. This can be done in a variety of ways—for example, having the clinician imitate the child, and the child imitate the clinician. Once the child is imitating what the clinician says and does, the clinician may begin to model single-word utterances for the child to imitate. This can be carried out in the context of a variety of such play activities as naming toy animals as they are put into the barn, naming puzzle pieces as they are put into place, or naming the actions performed by a puppet. Or, the clinician may leave the situation very fluid, and simply model the short utterances and by facial expression or gesture suggest that the child respond verbally.

Most children react well to the loose structure of the play situation, making it a favorable clinical setting. Although the clinician has specific goals to work on, the atmosphere at first is kept deliberately low key, and spontaneous speech is not aborted. A little later we will need more of that spontaneous speech to reinforce the child's newly acquired fluency and controls. Other methods of eliciting one-word utterance include asking either/or questions, asking yes/no questions, and having the child name pictures or objects. Most children are responsive to the less formal tasks. However, the clinician uses discretion and focuses at first on the method that will elicit the most fluency.

The clinician gradually begins to model longer utterances—two- and three-word phrases. That is, as the child begins to handle the smaller units fluently, the length of utterance is increased, still using short phrases or simple sentences—"A big cat," "He went in," "In the house," "Where is he?" "Here he is." Now the clinician elicits and encourages the same from the child.

If the young child is having difficulty with fluency on even small units of speech, the clinician may want to use additional fluency enhancers, such as talking with the child, and gradually fading her speech out as the child's fluency becomes more established. Attention to the physiological aspects of speech production may be warranted for the child who cannot be fluent on small linguistic units. For example, the clinician refers to "hard speech" and "easy speech" if the terms are considered to be appropriate for the child's level of awareness and sensitivity to stuttering. The methods used are those described under "The Physiological Factor," above. We have observed that the blocking is more likely to occur on the child's spontaneous insertions than on the somewhat controlled linguistic pattern that has been described. However, the child will walk out of the clinic and use the longer, spontaneous utterances; therefore we help him also to handle the results of those longer utterances, that is, the blocking.

The clinician meanwhile is continuing to increase the length of his or her utterances, and in time strings two clauses together to create an easy complex sentence. Similar sequencing of clauses may be required of the client by asking "And what happened then?" The clinician begins to make more demands of the child, requesting responses to questions that require longer, more complex answers, eliciting more complex picture descriptions, story telling, and conversational speech.

When the child is fluent or nearly so, and is able to use whatever has been taught in the way of controls, such as easy speech or cancellation, we begin to desensitize him or her to stress according to Van Riper's method with young stutterers. That is, we inject excitement into the play situation; we hurry and sometimes interrupt the child. Unlike Van Riper, we do not stop if we see the child about to stutter. If there is blocking, we simply help the child to use easy speech.

For the child who has a language lag, this method of sequencing the language units assures that the length and complexity of utterance can be kept within the client's capacity. In the early stages of therapy, while fluency and control are being established, the vocabulary should consist of words already in the child's lexicon. For the two-word stage, utterances comprised of familiar vocabulary may be used to facilitate fluency, while simultaneously reinforcing skill with the use of two word utterances. For example, if the child's vocabulary contains the words go, big, up, car, and boy, the structures "car go," "car up," "boy up," "boy go," "big car," and "big boy," may be created. Using appropriate toys, the clinician will find it a simple matter to elicit such structures in a limited play situation—(i.e., one that is confined by the materials the clinician chooses to have available to elicit and reinforce specific behaviors in the child). Gradually, new vocabulary may be added to the sessions to increase the child's repertoire. Similarly, new sentence structures may be added, keeping in mind the developmental sequence of the structures.

Although some language-delayed/fluency-disordered children go through this process smoothly, others experience ups and downs of fluency and disfluency. It is impossible to pinpoint the reasons for an increase in disfluency when the child has experienced a period of relative fluency. Some note the natural cyclicity of stuttering (see Van Riper's Track I description, 1971, 1982); others look for environmental influences. The children under discussion may seem to reach a point of wanting to communicate information that is cognitively beyond their linguistic capacity. This may also occur in children who seem to have been withholding speech, that is, have been communicating with relatively short, simple sentences and one-word responses, although giving the impression of having capacity beyond that. With more confidence in their verbal abilities, they may release the complexity that has been stored, but they are unable to cope physiologically with the results. These are speculations, however, and are yet to be verified. Usually the reappearance of disfluencies is temporary. It does not necessarily mean that the clinician is doing something "wrong," although certainly the sequencing and the pacing of the sessions should be evaluated.

The school-aged child usually can cope with quite direct attention to the stuttering. An exceptional case is the female stutterer mentioned previously, who had built up an array of antiexpectancy devices so strong that at first they acted as a "smoke screen," and the child kept the clinician at a distance from herself and her speech. Assuming that the child is cooperative, however, we use the child's spontaneous speech as much as possible as a tool in therapy. Also, because the older child is likely to be more at ease with questioning, we use questions to elicit one- and two-word responses. If the child cannot use two words without blocking, only one word is required. To do this work, the client is shown how to use loose contacts as well as slow-normal speech when giving responses to the questions. If the child seems to be embarrassed and self-conscious, the questions may be in the form of a word game. For instance: "I'm going to describe some objects in this room; you tell me what I'm talking about, using just one word. Don't forget your loose contacts." Questions should be innocuous, not designed to elicit stuttering, as in asking the child's name and address. Use neutral questions, such as "When do you get up in the morning?" "What's your favorite cereal?" or "Do you like the Mets or the Yankees?" Sometimes the child gives us a topic that is of interest, such as the Saturday baseball game, and we gear our questions to that. If the client blocks during responses, he or she is reminded to use loose contacts. Gradually the responses are built up to two- and three-word phrases and then short sentences. When longer sentences and complex sentences are required, conversation between the clinician and the client may be used to elicit the longer, more complex utterances. The clinician may ask "Why?" questions when the child is required to give a full (and complex) response. Picture descriptions and story telling are appropriate when the child can deal with longer utterances and use controls.

Some of the commercially available language kits offer suitable stimuli for school-aged children, and the level of complexity of the stimuli can be controlled—even to adding one morpheme at a time.

Dealing with Pragmatics

The adult stutterer is known to dilute the appropriateness of his language use at times by means of word substitutions and circumlocutions. This may apply, in varying degrees, to childhood stutterers. Although preschool children cannot participate in an objective discussion about this phenomenon, one need only observe the young child who falters in a sentence, inserts some "ums" or "ers," glances away, and produces a word that is out of context. It may happen rarely in a preschooler, and it may be more easily detected in looking at videotapes of the child, rather than during the interaction. It is possible for this to develop into a chronic habit by the time the child reaches high school or before; he or she may possess a repertoire of synonyms befitting the most mature stutterer, but interfering markedly with the appropriateness of conversation.

Because circumlocution seems to be a relatively undeveloped symptom in the preschooler, we do not work on it directly, assuming that the child's increasing confidence in the ability to talk will allow him to go ahead on any word. With the older child we are guided in our approach by the severity of the problem. For the milder cases, the avoidances may subside as the child gains increasing control over fluency and modification of blocks. For the more chronic cases, work on word avoidance is warranted when the child has some experience with fluency control and modification of the block. We ask such children to try to talk without switching words in a simple conversation with the clinician. Children who feel that they might stutter on an upcoming word are instructed to use loose contacts and to handle the word as easily as possible. They use hand counters to tally the number of substitutions or circumlocutions. We keep them talking until there is a substantial reduction of avoided words. Usually, client and clinician set a goal for success at the onset of the task, and work until the goal is met. We trust the integrity of our client in reporting avoided words to us, or, we give him or her the benefit of any doubt.

For the older and more severe stutterer, a concerted and organized Van Riperian effort may be necessary to desensitize the child to feared words and sounds, and to induce the child to implement the tools for fluency and modification of blocks on the feared stimuli.

The use of antiexpectancy devices also interferes with the appropriateness of the child's conversation. Frequent inappropriate laughter, for example, can be extremely disconcerting to the listener. There are, however, more subtle areas of pragmatics that may influence the fluency of the child on an individual basis. L. A. Nelson (1982) notes that children's disfluencies may increase "when they try to get us to listen to them, [because] they are not good at waiting their turn to talk." This is an example of increased disfluency when the child is in the "regulator" role (Bloom and Lahey, 1978). Guitar et al. (1981), in a single-subject study, found a high correlation between a verbal variable of "nonacceptingness" in the mother of a preschool stuttering child and the occurrence of secondary stuttering in the child. Individual patterns of reaction among child, parents, and others may be gleaned from the study of audio- or videotaped segments, and the situations can then be used to help to generalize the child's control or modification of stuttering to the "difficult" situations;

that is, the situations are simulated in the therapy session and the child is encouraged to use easy speech or loose contacts while participating.

Summary

When the psycholinguistic factor is stressed, the child's fluency is enhanced in a linguistically controlled, low structured setting. The clinician uses a slow-normal speech rate and, having a choice of several techniques, elicits short utterances from the child. The length of utterance is gradually increased if the child is mostly fluent. If the child does not achieve fluency at even the one- and two-word level, the clinician may use simultaneous speech, gradually fading out. Alternatively, reference to the physiological aspects of production—hard versus easy speech—may help the child to modify the blocks.

There is a continued but gradual increase in the length of utterance required of the child, with a continuation of easy speech, and introduction of techniques to modify blocks as necessary—loose contacts, and simple versions of pullouts and cancellations. With increased fluency and control of stuttering, the child is desensitized to excitement, hurry, and interruption, and is encouraged to use fluency and controls in such situations.

Special vocabulary and semantic-syntactic adaptation are made for the child with a language delay. New sentence structures introduced should adhere to the developmental sequence of language.

For the school-aged stutterer, easy speech using loose contacts and slow-normal rate are incorporated into increased length of utterance. A variety of techniques may be used to elicit the graduated utterances—questions and answers, word games, a language kit, simple conversation. Techniques for modifying the blocks are incorporated into the fluency enhancement sequencing of increasing linguistic units. Eventually the child should be using fluency and controls for complex language tasks such as picture descriptions and conversation, and for complex responses to the clinician's questions.

Pragmatic appropriateness is increased for all children by decreasing word substitution and circumlocution, as well as by increasing the pragmatic repertoire of the child while maintaining fluency.

Table 3 summarizes therapies according to our three-factor framework.

CONCLUSION

Generalization of Fluency and Controls

With preschool children the generalization of fluency and control of the blocks sometimes takes place spontaneously. This is our observation and

Table 3. Summary of therapy according to the three factors

Psychosocial factor	Physiological factor	Psycholinguistic factor
For the child	For the child	For the child
Increase fluency Slow-normal speech rate Acknowledge "hard" versus "easy" speech	*Increase fluency* Slow-normal speech rate Use easy speech	*Increase fluency* Slow-normal speech rate Easy speech on controlled linguistic units
For child's reaction to speech Reduce avoidances—sound, word, situation Deal with others' reactions to stuttering Increase child's self-esteem	*Respiration* Use appropriate pause time Correct aberrant patterns	*Extend linguistic units according to semantic-syntactic level* Utterances 1-2 word long Utterances 3-4 word long Increase the length Increase the complexity Conjoin clauses
For Parents and Significant Others	*Phonation* Easy onsets for voice and speech Easy speech Coordinate respiration and phonation	*Increase linguistic demands of child* In response to questions In conversational speech Other linguistic tasks
Counsel regarding Stuttering (general information) Stuttering moments Language and speech acquisition Parental language complexity Environmental fluency disrupters Familial/child adjustment	*Coarticulation* Loose contacts Pullouts Cancellation	*Attention to pragmatics* Examples: Turn taking in conversation Appropriate eye contact (Adapt as necessary for the child with language-speech delay)
	Associated symptoms Behavior modification techniques as necessary	
	Generalization Child uses fluency and controls in varied situations and with varied people	

that of others (Adams, 1980; Ryan, 1979; Shine, 1980). If spontaneous generalization does not occur, we bring family members into the session and accustom the child to using the new skill in their presence. Other clinicians and clients of similar age are recruited to share activities and discourse. The child is taken out to work on speech while talking with the clinician over a soda, or during a game of ball on the lawn. That is, we vary the people, and we vary the physical environment as much as possible, so that speech skills are reinforced in a variety of contexts. This is in addition, or course, to generalization activities noted for the more subtle pragmatic events.

For the older child, the feared situations in the hierarchy previously mentioned serve as generalization activities. In addition, we vary the people with whom the child talks, and the situational context of the conversations, as for the younger stutterers. One of the most important activities for the school-aged child may be having him or her use the new skills in the class. It is certainly advisable to gain the support and cooperation of the classroom teacher by discussing the child's progress from time to time. Any particularly difficult assignment that the child may have been avoiding at school, such as an oral report, may prove to be an ideal activity. We have sometimes spent a lot of therapy time simulating the classroom and giving the child rehearsal time in front of an audience, before the child embarks on the actual assignment. In addition, however, we make sure that our client is still aware of the range of choices regarding speech production. Assuming that the goal for the presentation to the class is slow-normal speech rate and loose contacts (not abnormally loose), the child still has pullouts and cancellation as backup systems if necessary. Occasional reminders of the choices are also reminders of the control over the speech pattern that the child has gained.

Discharge and Followup

As a guideline for clinicians who require a percentage of stutterings as a criterion for discharge, we recommend the use of Ryan's (1979) 0.4% disfluency or less when remaining stutterings are counted, and Webster's (1979) 3% or less when *all* nonfluencies (remaining mild stutterings plus normal nonfluencies) are counted. When the child has experienced fluency within normal limits, for 2 to 3 months, the maintenance phase of therapy is begun. If the new fluency pattern is to stay, it must be firmly reinforced. In addition to such fluency, the child should have stopped avoiding speech situations and should feel comfortable with most speaking situations. We see the child for a followup appointment 2 months later, scheduling two more such followups, and then a visit every 6 months, until the client has remained fluent for approximately 2 years. We emphasize, however, that parents should contact us any time they wish to discuss a problem.

Home Practice

We are not as rigid about home practice as many clinicians. If we feel that home practice is not advisable for some reason, we do not institute it. For example, home practice might be contraindicated in a family where both parents work and an atmosphere of "busyness" prevails to the extent that further involvement of the parents, except on an informal and casual level, is not appropriate. In such a case we might encourage the child to accomplish certain goals, and alert the parents to the goals so that they can facilitate their achievement. We like to have even quite young children accept responsibility for "carryover" as soon as possible. A clinician may exclaim to a 5-year-old who is moving well through therapy: "Wow, I love that easy speech you're using. How about trying it out tonight when you and mommy read to each other, and let me know next time how it worked out." The clinician would follow up at the next session, asking if the child had accomplished the goal. Although attitudes may change during therapy, and adjustments for home practice may occur accordingly, as a general rule parents who are already excessively critical of the child's performance would not be asked to do unsupervised work with the child.

For the younger child, the parents' less direct help as described in connection with the psychosocial factor of therapy usually suffices. However, through parental observation of therapy sessions with young children, and through counseling, the parents may also learn to talk and play with their youngster in a way that promotes fluency: that is, the parents may learn to reduce their utterances during play and have a very relaxed, shared time with their child when speech is slow and easy.

We use home practice for the older child, always ensuring that the task prescribed for home practice is a little below the level of the one being worked on clinically. This ensures that the child will be able to perform appropriately, and further difficulties will not be created by the parent helping the child with something that is too advanced.

The Gestalt of Therapy

Therapy from the three factors is integrated into a whole. Work with the parents proceeds as work with the child simultaneously takes place. Modification techniques, which are subsumed under "physiological" aspects of stuttering, are integrated with the fluency-enhancing techniques described in the section on the psycholinguistic factor. Slow-normal speech rate and loose contacts are clearly fundamental features of therapy and may be quite powerful when used with the fluency-enhancing techniques of increased length and complexity of utterance. Further modification techniques, however, probably will be necessary for the more severe stutterer. Again, psychosocial, physiological, and psycholinguistic techniques should be selected to dovetail with the diagnostic profile presented at the evaluation, or developed over time spent with the child and the family. Not all techniques are intended for every child stutterer.

The Making of a Therapy

Therapy is a process that evolves over time; it does not appear as an inspiration to a select clinician. Therapies are built on the strengths of previous therapies, placed in the context of new information, and often in the context of a thoughtful and creative clinician. The overlap that exists in the therapies presented in the preceding chapter, and with our own therapy, is quite proper. Our therapy draws heavily on many of Van Riper's techniques, and on recent information in the fields of psycholinguistics, developmental psycholinguistics, and the physiology of speech production. It differs from the current programmed techniques for fluency shaping in that we use both fluency-enhancing techniques and modification techniques; in addition, we use a low structured situation with the young child, and we place more responsibility on the clinician for goal setting and selection of stimuli, hence greater flexibility and allowance for creativity. We do not regard one way or the other as "better." In fact we sometimes switch a client from a looser structure to a tighter one, if we think it is right for that individual. This is an important point, that the clinician be flexible enough to make a change for the client's benefit. Ryan and Van Kirk (1978) presumably had this in mind when they designed "branching steps" for their program; this provides some flexibility in the program.

The Unwilling Client

Even when one has decided on a treatment approach that makes sense, some children who are presented for therapy seem to be unwilling or unable to participate in the nicely ordered approach that the clinician has developed. This may be because the child does not want to be there, with you, working on speech. It does not mean that the child does not want his or her speech to get better. However, the child may not want to have anything to do with the process of getting it better. This is particularly likely to occur with the school-aged stutterer, when the clinician's best efforts may be met with sullen resistance. Individual clinicians develop their own styles of dealing with this kind of child. We have found that trying to talk the client out of his or her point of view is a great "turn-off." We never try to argue a child out of reactions or to make the child "see reason." Frequently it is helpful to empathize briefly and simply—"It must be a pain being somewhere that you don't want to be. I know you'd rather be out with your friends, right? Let's get to work and when we're through you can get back to them." Some children are responsive to the invitation to bring a best friend to therapy; others abhor the idea. Some young clients "thaw out" and begin to verbalize more freely if the clinician involves them in physical activities, such as a miniature bowling game or constructing with building blocks, simply talking along while playing, rather than quizzing them about themselves and their stuttering. Such activities can also lead to work on stuttering, and in time most children can be channeled into productive speech work.

The Clinician and the Programs

Many school clinicians have adopted therapy programs for use with stutterers, apparently in an effort to accommodate the "accountability" issue in the schools, to simplify the acquisition of quantifiable data for the individualized education plans (IEP's) and, in some instances, to obtain a cohesive therapy approach with child stutterers. These reasons are plausible. Most clinicians recognize, however, that if the goal is to collect 10 fluent one-word utterances from a 5-year-old, it does not matter whether client and clinician are engaged in informal play or seated at a table, with the child requested to name 10 pictures and be fluent. Clinicians recognize that even if they choose programmed therapy, they are not exempt from thinking about the individual needs of their small clients. Applying programs across the spectrum of clients without thought gives rise to the complaint "But it doesn't always work." Although we have many techniques that are frequently highly effective with stutterers, it is certainly hard to produce a package of them that will "always work." It is up to the clinician to be aware of available alternatives and to use them appropriately. Many school clinicians now use manuals that outline steps for the treatment of various speech, language, and voice disorders. The presentation of material in the manual facilitates the writing of IEP's for the clinician. One such manual is by N. W. Nelson (1979). Some steps from a program for use with school-aged stutterers appear below. The goal for this program is: "The student will speak in all situations with no more than normal dysfluencies." The long-range objective is: "The student will speak fluently in conversation for five minutes with no stuttered words." Assume that Stage 1 "stretch and flow," has been carried out successfully, and the client moves on to Stage 2, "increased breath."

1. *Continue using appropriate relaxation.*
2. *Increase the rate of speech while maintaining excessive breathiness, low intensity, relative monotone, and loose articulation when instructed to talk using Stage 2 style.*
3. *Demonstrate the use of fluent Stage 2 speech in at least three*

low stress situations outside the clinic room on three different days.

4. *Talk using Stage 2 style without interferences during timed observations of reading, monologue and dialogue (three minutes each on two different days)*

(N. W. Nelson, 1979, pp. 205–206).

An example of a branching step for this program might be an intermediary goal between step 2 and step 3, if our imaginary child in therapy is unable to carry out effectively step 3. The branching step might read: "Demonstrate the use of fluent Stage 2 speech in the clinic room in low stress conditions." That is, the level of difficulty has been reduced by switching the locale from the more threatening outside situation to the therapy room. Simple adjustments to a program may make the difference between a child experiencing failure and success, and his individual needs will have been met.

Although the clinician may feel secure using one particular therapy with all children who stutter, success as a clinician may ultimately depend on the clinician's ability to make informed decisions about which route to take in therapy (be it creating a branching step for a program, or instituting intensive parent counseling). To some extent this ability comes with experience, but it is also a very important function of knowledge of one's field, personal maturity, and flexibility.

Case History Presentations

The case presentations that follow have been selected to help illustrate therapy with the preschool child. The evaluation data on Robert in Figure 2 are set out according to the three-factor model.

Case 1. Robert

At evaluation Robert had stuttered for almost a year; the symptoms had worsened considerably. Associated symptoms, such as hair pulling (Figure 2), were recent. Because the boy seemed to withhold speech at the evaluation, the spontaneous speech sample on which data on stuttering were based was obtained on his first and second therapy sessions. Therapy was scheduled on a trial basis of one hourly session per week. Robert's progress was satisfactory, no increase in weekly sessions was necessary.

The Therapy

● *Sessions 1 and 2*   The clinician aimed to establish rapport with Robert, in a low structured setting, and to elicit a spontaneous language sample to be audiotaped for an analysis of MLU and stuttering. The two talked

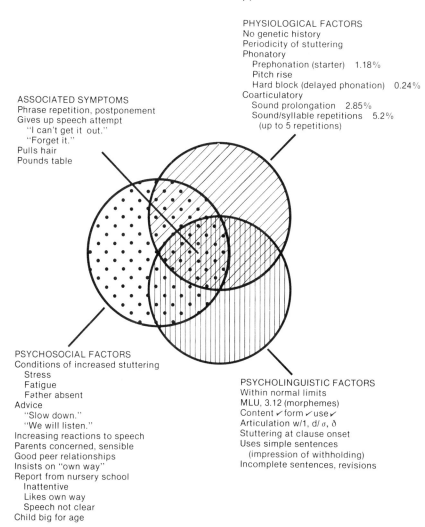

PHYSIOLOGICAL FACTORS
No genetic history
Periodicity of stuttering
Phonatory
    Prephonation (starter)   1.18%
    Pitch rise
    Hard block (delayed phonation)   0.24%
Coarticulatory
    Sound prolongation   2.85%
    Sound/syllable repetitions   5.2%
    (up to 5 repetitions)

ASSOCIATED SYMPTOMS
Phrase repetition, postponement
Gives up speech attempt
    "I can't get it out."
    "Forget it."
Pulls hair
Pounds table

PSYCHOSOCIAL FACTORS
Conditions of increased stuttering
    Stress
    Fatigue
    Father absent
Advice
    "Slow down."
    "We will listen."
Increasing reactions to speech
Parents concerned, sensible
Good peer relationships
Insists on "own way"
Report from nursery school
    Inattentive
    Likes own way
    Speech not clear
Child big for age

PSYCHOLINGUISTIC FACTORS
Within normal limits
MLU, 3.12 (morphemes)
Content ✓ form ✓ use ✓
Articulation w/1, d/ σ, ð
Stuttering at clause onset
Uses simple sentences
    (impression of withholding)
Incomplete sentences, revisions

Figure 2. Evaluation data for Robert, aged 3 years, 10 months; syllables stuttered, 9.5%.

together while playing; the clinician did not attempt to limit Robert's utterances because she wanted spontaneity for the analyses. Nevertheless, he kept utterances short, made frequent use of one-word utterances, and frequently failed to complete what he wanted to say. He also deflected involvement in some activities with "I don't wanna" and "You do it." He went out to check on his mother twice during the first session. Associated physical symptoms (hair pulling, foot stamping) were not exhibited at this or subsequent sessions.

• *Session 3*   The aims were for the clinician to use slow-normal speech rate and simple speech constructions as a model for Robert, to encourage Robert to do the same, to help him to complete some unfinished sentences (even if stuttering was incurred), and to draw attention at least once to "hard" speech. Limiting Robert's sentences was simplified by his own tendency to use utterances about three words long. When the clinician commented that a prolongation "sounded a bit hard" he glanced at her and went on playing. When she suggested that he complete some statements, he complied.

• *Session 4*   The aims were as for Session 3. The client exhibited prolongations of sounds and syllabic/sound repetitions. He was not responsive to the clinician's offer to help him say a word over again "the easy way." He completed all utterances that he began without incurring more stuttering. The overall rate of stuttering was reduced as compared with preceding sessions, and there were still no signs of physical associated behaviors.

• *Session 5 to 7*   Aims were for fluent utterances of moderate length and attention to "hard" blocks when they occurred. The short sentences were encouraged, but longer utterances were not aborted. About twice in each session, the clinician casually commented "Oh, that looked hard to say." Once Robert replied that he had to go, although he didn't leave. In another instance the clinician encouraged Robert to say something over the easy way because "The turtle didn't hear you." He complied. A jointed "scarecrow" and puppets were introduced to demonstrate floppy, relaxed limbs. The scarecrow or puppets demonstrated relaxed, loose, easy speech, which Robert was encouraged to use. By now Robert was more at ease and frequently avoided completion of tasks by saying "I'll do it later." This was similar to the mother's complaint that he "likes his own way."

• *Session 8*   Robert now exhibited a decrease in disfluencies in the clinic and the same was reported at home; body movements had totally subsided without any direct therapeutic attention; speech was generally easier, and Robert was rarely giving up the speech attempt and rarely incurring a hard block.

The aims now were to elicit longer, more complex language, and to focus more on "cancellation" of hard blocks or noticeable prolongations and repetitions. Also, Robert's nursery school was concerned about his visual-motor skills, and some tasks involving these skills were introduced. He was totally uninterested in such tasks and unwilling to engage in any cutting or pencil-and-paper activities.

Still using the low structured setting, which sometimes involved activities such as making Playdoh to create objects, the clinician encouraged Robert's use of longer utterances and connected utterances. By this time he was willing to repeat some stuttered words over the "easy" way, but he did this at the clinician's request, not spontaneously. The clinician found that Robert was uncomfortable with visual-motor activities. He thought he wasn't good at them and had little confidence in his attempts. She adjusted tasks to give him success.

Pragmatic aspects of communication were also attended to at this time. Robert's turn-taking reaction of "You do it" or "I'll do mine later" was less acceptable to the clinician, and Robert responded more appropriately.

● *Session 10*   As for Session 8, with mild desensitization procedures included. The clinician talked faster, quickened the pace of the session, and occasionally attempted to hurry Robert or to interrupt him. He maintained a calm attitude and his speech was not disrupted. At this time he was still completing all sentences, and remaining fluent or almost fluent for long sentences.

The client was then absent during a 5-week semester break. Upon return Robert exhibited four instances of sound prolongation and two instances of word repetition in an hour of free play and spontaneous conversation. The clinician asked if he had remembered to use his easy speech, he replied "Yeah, I guess so." The goals of therapy were readjusted to the reinforcement of fluency and the remediation of defective sounds L and TH, beginning with L. In addition, continued help with visual-motor coordination was deemed advisable.

● *Session 12*   During play and free conversation, the clinician occasionally asked "Are you using your easy speech?" as a reminder. When a minor disfluency occurred (there were no major disfluencies), she cautioned, "Easy, Robert." He responded well and appeared to loosen up deliberately. He spontaneously repeated (or "canceled") some disfluent words at this time in the clinic and at home.

Work on L words proceeded smoothly; the work was incorporated into Robert's play activities. He was beginning to take pride in completing pencil-and-paper tasks such as coloring and connecting-the-dots pictures.

● *Session 14*   Robert was reacting well to reminders to use his easy speech. He occasionally loosened his articulators and eased out of a repetition, as though gliding over the disruptions.

● *Session 16*   Fluency was consistent, with only occasional minor interruptions, which Robert handled well. He was using long and complex utterances, as well as complex words—brontosaurus, ankylosaurus. The L sound was becoming stabilized in general speech patterns.

No formal work was done on associated symptoms except for encouraging Robert to complete utterances; the associated symptoms spontaneously subsided. Generalization of fluency and control also occurred spontaneously, although the clinician sometimes asked Robert if he had been using his "easy speech" at home, and further indirect methods of help at home were discussed with the parents.

● *Additional Sessions*   Although Robert was usually fluent at this stage of therapy, he attended for another 10 weeks so that his fluency could be reinforced and his newly acquired sounds stabilized. Perhaps we err on the side of caution in prolonging therapy in this way, but we want the child to communicate with maximum efficiency, and some past experiences with relapse encourage us to be cautious.

Parent Counseling   Both Robert's parents attended hour-long sessions at the onset of therapy. The mother then attended four sessions, and thereafter was seen monthly or as necessary. The main focus of the early sessions was the parents' concern with how to react to the stuttering, and how to promote more fluency in Robert's speech. Because the child reacted well to their encouragement to "slow down" and their reassurance that "we will listen," and they were comfortable with this method, it was suggested that they continue with it. Later, when the mother had observed therapy by closed-circuit video several times, she became sensitive to "hard" and "easy" speech, and occasionally used a phrase like "that looked hard to say" when Robert was having a difficult time with the blocking. She was counseled to use this method sparingly. She was also counseled to use slower speech. In addition, suggestions were made to reduce linguistic demands, particularly during periods of fatigue and excitement. Ways in which the mother might increase the child's sense of ease and security when the father was away from home were discussed, because the stuttering worsened during these absences.

Through discussion and observing therapy, Robert's mother gained insights into how she might use her own language in talking to Robert to facilitate his more fluent speech production. She was also able to discuss her concern about the blocking when it occurred.

A nursery school aide had commented negatively about Robert's behavior and speech and, with the parents' permission, we contacted the school. The complaints were about generally poor communication (Robert hung his head and spoke indistinctly when approached by the aide), and poor concentration. We tracked the "poor concentration" to the specific tasks of visual-motor coordination. Therapy was adjusted to help him with visual-motor work, at the same time pointing out to his mother and the nursery school that he was quite young (although his size made him look a good 2 years older) and had time to develop these skills. The school report also prompted us to begin work on Roberts articulatory difficulties.

This child's environment was a warm and loving one. The concern initially expressed by the parents was appropriate. Through their insistence, the pediatrician had referred them for help. When we began therapy, the stuttering was still cyclic, but becoming more consistent, and Robert exhibited strong reactions. We believe that this child probably avoided becoming a persistent stutterer because of the early referral.

Followup Telephone conversations with Robert's mother 2 and 4 months after discharge revealed that the client had maintained his gains. For a variety of domestic reasons his reevaluation at the clinic was deferred for a year. At the time of the reevaluation Robert, now 5.5 years old, interacted appropriately with the clinician, all aspects of language use were within normal limits, and fluency was normal. During 50 minutes of play and talking there were two minor disruptions that were considered to be within normal limits. Robert's mother reported fluent, intelligible speech in all situations. She also viewed him as a healthy, responsive child who was handling social, home, and school situations well.

Case 2. John

This case, still in progress, is presented because it exemplifies some fairly routine therapeutic anomalies: for instance, a child who acts appropriately at the evaluation but has difficulty in participating in therapy; a parent who becomes skeptical about therapy when the child's fluency improves in the clinic but shows little change "outside." At evaluation, John, aged 4.5 years, was reported to have stuttered since age 3. The parents were concerned but tried to follow the pediatrician's advice to ignore the problem. During the intervening 18 months the condition changed from episodic to consistent stuttering. Physical struggle, extended repetitions and prolongations, and various manifestations of more advanced stuttering accumulated. The parents eventually sought referral from the pediatrician because the child's nursery school teacher reported that his voluntary attempts to answer questions in school were "pitiful." She described prolonged struggle in his attempts to get speech started and urged the parents to seek help. A taped sample of John's spontaneous speech revealed a high rate of stuttering—16% of syllables were stuttered. According to John's mother, who was present when the child's speech was taped, the sample accurately represented the frequency of his stuttering in other situations, but not the severity (length and struggle) of the blocks.

At the beginning of therapy the family consisted of the client, an 8-year-old brother, an infant sister, and the parents. Further discussion is organized according to psychosocial, physiological, and psychological factors.

The Psychosocial Factor At the onset of therapy, there was some strain in the household because the family of five lived in a modest-sized apartment. In addition, the father was temporarily engaged in long hours of work on many days of the week and could spend little time with his family. Both parents were young and took their family and work responsibilities quite seriously.

The mother expressed her extreme distress at the severe stuttering of her middle child; the father was less affected, but recently had had minimal contact with John. When the stuttering was severe, the parents told John to take his time, otherwise they ignored it. The older brother frequently told John "If you can't say it, shut up." The parents noted that excitement exacerbated the stuttering.

John was reported to want to talk, stutter or not, and loved to do so even in what seemed to be his most difficult situations—discussion in the classroom and on class trips. He always persisted with speech in those situations, but sometimes gave up the speech attempt in other situations. He told his parents "It [speech] gets stuck in my throat." Although John seemed mature and independent at the evaluation, and the parents spoke of him in these terms, they later described "willful" behavior at home, and occasional tantrums when he did not get his way. He played alone at home for the most part; sometimes with his brother. The parents did not spend any time with John individually and commented that he preferred to play alone.

The Physiological Factor   John's birth, development, and health history were reported to be within normal limits. The maternal uncle was a severe, untreated stutterer. The physiological features of John's stuttering were as follows.

Respiration. Some talking on inhalation and occasional slight gasping for breath prior to speech.

Phonation. Frequent use of prephonation—an elongated vowel—as a starter; it sometimes changed to vocal fry and sometimes incorporated unsuccessful articulatory attempts to move into speech; hard blocks (silent pauses) with delayed phonation and struggle to phonate.

Coarticulation. Sound and syllable repetitions (up to four per block) and prolongations prevented smooth transitional movements.

Other physiological concomitants of stuttering included facial and jaw movements in attempts to emit speech, some eye closure, and arm movements used as a starting device.

The Psycholinguistic Factor   The client's language and speech use was within normal limits (MLU 5.8 morphemes). Sentences were frequently left incomplete and then revised. The prephonation of elongated vowels was usually, but not totally, attributable to John's difficulty in getting started at sentence or clause onsets with the words "I" and "and." The appropriateness of his verbal interaction was good at the evaluation; later in therapy sessions this area was deemed inconsistently satisfactory for his age.

Two hour-long therapy sessions per week were scheduled for John. A primarily language-based approach was planned, as for Robert (Case 1), with physiological and psychosocial aspects of therapy incorporated.

The Therapy

• *Sessions 1 to 4*   The aims of therapy were to establish rapport and to facilitate fluency in interactive play. The clinician planned to use short utterances with slow-normal rate, and to elicit the same from John. Although appropriate toys were available and the situation seemed to be nonthreatening, John could interact for only 2 or 3 minutes at a time. He then insisted on playing alone. In the brief periods of interaction the limited utterances he used in response to the clinician's encouragement or modeling were fluent. His extended utterances during parallel play, when the clinician also played and talked, were highly stuttered. On the fourth session there was an unfortunate but unavoidable change of clinician.

• *Session 5*   The new clinician attempted an interactional situation with a turn-taking activity. John was oppositional and refused to participate. His protests were loud and the situation provoked a high level of stuttering. The clinician reverted to parallel play, where the client felt more comfortable and in control. Later they returned successfully to interactive play and turn taking when a food reward was used. This time the situation did not provoke a high rate of stuttering; calm prevailed and short, fluent utterances of two and three words were elicited.

• *Sessions 6 to 9*   The goal was introducing "hard" versus "easy" speech, for severe blocks only. John sometimes nodded his head to "That looked hard to say," and inconsistently complied by following the clinician's model when she stated "Let me show you an easier way to say that." Brief (4- and 5-minute) periods of interactive play were interspersed with longer periods of parallel play. Turn-taking activities such as putting puzzle pieces together, and picture matching, were introduced, to elicit short, fluent phrases such as "This goes here," "Put that there," and "This is Snoopy." By the ninth session the client's attitude was less guarded and there was more sharing of activities. At this time John's mother reported that the child was occasionally stopping in his conversation to go back and repeat a "hard" word fluently, that is, he spontaneously canceled a stuttered word. The older brother visited the clinic during one of these sessions and observed part of his brother's therapy with the supervising clinician. He expressed some of his angry reactions to his brother's stuttered speech and, after discussion, agreed to try to stop telling John to "shut up" when he stuttered. He then joined the clinician and John in therapy for the last part of the session because we wanted him to feel involved in the therapy. We followed up later to note his further reactions to the stuttering.

● *Sessions 10 to 12*   John was now happy to consistently imitate the clinician's easy modeled utterances and to effect changes on most of his hard stuttered speech. Of seven hard blocks in one session, he successfully canceled five with clinician cuing of "That looked hard to say." He nodded his head in agreement that it was hard, then repeated the utterance easily and fluently. In addition, longer fluent utterances were encouraged in play, where interactive skills were progressing, but were still below the level that we hoped for.

● *Sessions 13 to 19*   The aims were still to facilitate fluency, to encourage self-correction of hard blocks, and to increase interactive abilities. John had six hard blocks in the first of these sessions—three that the clinician helped him to correct and three that he corrected to her cuing. He accepted an increasingly direct approach to his speech. For example, the clinician said, "Try not to push when you say it." John answered, "OK." Or again, "That time you didn't push when you said it." "Right." And "Your talking has been nice and easy today." "Thank you." At this time the clinician could cue John to correct by placing her hand on his arm. The client was now interacting with the clinician for approximately 75% of each session.

● *Sessions 20 to 23*   An added aim was to confront John more directly when he was oppositional. When he refused to participate the clinician might remark, good-naturedly, "You're so bossy today!" or "You certainly want your own way today!" There were increasing signs of his flexibility, however, and of his growing willingness to compromise rather than provoke an argument or a standoff. At this time (10 weeks into therapy), a tape-recorded sample of John's speech during a clinical session (consisting of a mixture of free play and talk with some fluency-enhancing conditions and controlled linguistic units incorporated) revealed a stuttering rate of 4.1%. (See the parent counseling section of this case report for contrasting rates of stuttering.)

● *Sessions 24 to 27*   Mild desensitization procedures were introduced to the clinical setting. A little excitement was injected into the play, toy telephones were used for telephone practice, and "show and tell" activities were attempted. Excitement did not disturb John's fluency in this setting, nor did the telephone activity. John limited his show and tell activities to singing songs, however, and at this time refused to introduce variety into the situation. The final session of this group, John had been told, would be his last for a short while because it was the end of the semester. Stuttering increased in this session, and John needed clinician help in modeling and cuing to regain his former fluency. He was reassured about the resumption of therapy in the near future.

• *Sessions 27 to 37*   The next 10 sessions were with a new clinician, to whom John adjusted quickly. The clinician reinforced John's fluency in sentences ranging from long (five and six words) simple sentences to sentences of roughly equivalent length but syntactically more complex. This was done primarily through the use of a language kit, and partially through the child's participation in games. The clinician continued the work of encouraging his interaction during the session, and on one occasion when she did not specifically engage him, he asked "Could I play with you?" The clinician made demands of him to stick to the rules of the games they played instead of making up his own rules. He complied and remained fluent except for an occasional word repetition, rather than a disintegration of fluency, which had been his former response to this kind of request. The clinician initiated a discussion with John on relaxation and easy speech, which he effectively "tuned out" in the early part of their relationship but accepted with apparent interest during the last therapy session. He helped to construct a book in which speakers were depicted in various states of ease or tension. He and the clinician discussed who, of the speakers, was talking "easy" and who was talking "hard." The book was to serve as a visual reminder of easy and hard speech during the summer break. At this point in his sessions, John experienced only occasional and mild disfluencies, which he corrected.

John reached an important milestone related to the generalization of fluency in these last 5 weeks of therapy. Although his stuttering had reduced in outside situations, there had not been complete generalization. He went on a school trip, however, and typically he wanted to participate in a discussion. His old struggle began and no words emerged. His teacher came to his side and said "Easy, John," at which time he visibly relaxed, composed himself, and made his comment fluently to the group. In addition, John's mother reported that he was fluent for most of each day, appearing to "glide" through any small blocks that came along. The stuttering returned, not in its severe form but certainly in mild to moderate form, at the end of the day when he was tired.

Parent Counseling   Both parents were seen for an initial discussion about John's stuttering. Thereafter the mother was seen weekly for 2 months and then intermittently. Both parents were seen to discuss progress before the summer break. Only the most salient counseling points of this case are discussed, because many more general points covered were discussed in Robert's (Case 1) therapy. John's parents were attuned to the importance of their own language use on the child's fluency. For example, the mother stopped questioning him about events in school when he arrived home each afternoon because these questions had precipitated a high rate of stuttering. It was suggested that she might comment "You look as though you enjoyed (or did not enjoy) yourself today" and leave any other conversation up to him. Or, she might greet him and say nothing about school. She later reported that John, having had an after-school refreshment, would spontaneously come to her to report the day's activities without the severe struggle her questioning had triggered.

It was also suggested that the parents take time out to play and to talk individually with John. This fell largely to the mother, but the father also tried. The mother began to spend about half an hour a day with John playing, reading, and looking at picture books. She observed therapy and noted ways in which the clinician promoted more fluency in this type of situation. She proved to be an effective fluency facilitator. Her reports and a tape recording reflected not only John's more fluent speech, but his apparent appreciation of spending this unhurried time with his mother.

Two months after the onset of therapy, John's stuttering had decreased noticeably in the clinic, but the mother, observing therapy, assured us that his speech was "much worse" in outside situations than in the clinic. We reassured her that it was appropriate for his gains to be manifested clinically at first and that he would be helped to generalize these gains to outside situations. Nevertheless, we were curious about the severity of his stuttering in other situations and asked her to tape record the child's speech, if possible, in a variety of situations. Within the same week, we collected a sample of spontaneous speech from the therapy session which, as previously noted, consisted of some speech when fluency was facilitated, and some when there was free play and free talk with moderate excitement. The rate of stuttering in the clinical situation was 4.1% of syllables; in a quiet talking period at home with his mother, 7%; and in a "stress situation, 15%. The stress situation consisted of a conversation at a ballgame where there was considerable background noise and activity; John was talking with a linguistically demanding adult, a fast speaker who bombarded the child with information and questions, frequently interrupting him with another thought or question. A similarly high rate of stuttering was noted, however, for a situation that involved John's attempting to ask his mother important questions while she was attending to the baby. The content of the tapes became useful in the counseling sessions, and was helpful as we proceeded to plan some desensitization procedure for John's sessions.

Although the client's mother acknowledged that he needed his own way fairly frequently and that there were sometimes tantrums when he did not get it, she felt that she and her husband handled the situations calmly and well. We did not, therefore, make suggestions in that area or suggest an alternate form of counseling, but told her that we would like to have John's participation in some activities and that we were working to get it.

Because John showed gradual improvement and increased flexibility in his verbal interactions, we became less concerned about this area.

There were three telephone contacts with the teacher, who was an experienced and sensible person. She became a valuable ally in the generalization of fluency, as the anecdote of the class trip illustrates. The parents also became adept at helping John to loosen up. It was very hard for the mother to do this at first, however, because she was afraid of making her son more self-conscious and worsening the condition. In addition, she was nonplussed by the child's response the first time she commented that "That looked hard to say." He replied, with some disgust, "Of course it was hard to say. That's why I couldn't say it!"

Followup   John's therapy was interrupted at this point, after 4.5 months because of the summer break. Reevaluation was scheduled for the fall, with therapy plans to be devised according to the results of that evaluation.

Case 3.   Adam

> Adam's stuttering symptoms at evaluation (age 4.5 years) were judged to be moderate. The beginning stuttering was reported to be episodic, exhibiting silent blocks with minimal force or tension. Shortly before coming for an evaluation, however, Adam's mother had observed facial contortions with mouth opening as if waiting for a word to come out. Adam did not evidence frustration or avoidance of speaking situations. During the diagnostic session, Adam's symptoms included silent blocks, which varied in degree of force and tension, occasional eye closure, and intermittent vowel glides in an attempt to come out of a block. Except for the possibility of an occasional word avoidance, Adam did not seem to be concerned or frustrated, even though his parents had told him the reason ("difficulty with speech") for coming to the clinic. Family history revealed that a maternal cousin and a paternal nephew had stuttered but that both had outgrown the symptoms.

The Psychosocial Factor   The family seemed to be a very warm and loving unit, and the household presented itself as being very talkative, self-expressive, and open. The maternal grandparents spoke consistently in Italian to Adam, and referred to Adam's speech difficulty as "this problem," or "this poor boy." Other family members spoke about Adam's stuttering in his presence. Adam's father on occasion asked Adam to "talk perfectly or don't talk." Moreover, the parental speech rate was very rapid. The mother reported that Adam and his younger brother continually vied for attention, particularly from the father, who worked long hours at his carpentry business.

The Physiological Factor   Adam's medical history was unremarkable except for frequent colds, ear infections, and upper respiratory infections. It was observed that Adam's general level of activity and even his level of disfluency were heightened on days when he received medication for the infections. As mentioned in the beginning of the case history, family history revealed that a maternal cousin and a paternal nephew had stuttered. We also observed an occasional high degree of disfluencies in Adam's younger brother toward the middle of the therapy year.

The Psycholinguistic Factor   Adam's speech and language milestones were within normal limits. His mother provided a great deal of language stimulation at home when he was younger. Adam exhibited a wide variety of appropriate pragmatic functions and engaged in many interactions not only with family members but also with peers at his nursery school.

The Therapy

● *Sessions 1 to 4*   The initial sessions aimed to establish rapport and to continue collecting baseline data on Adam. In addition to the characteristics noted during the diagnostic session, Adam exhibited prolongations on such words as "what," "you," and "I" and occasionally used starter phrases such as "I think." His disfluencies from the beginning were less on utterances that were syntactically, semantically, and pragmatically simpler.

● *Sessions 5 to 9*   After observing a core set of baseline behaviors, the clinician began to facilitate an awareness of "hard" (disfluent) and "soft" (fluent) speech by clinician modeling and playback of clinician's speech from the tape recorder. At the same time, fluency-enhancing contexts were created whereby the linguistic load placed on Adam was relatively undemanding. The nature of the therapy activities ranged from relatively structured and simple activities such as describing pictures and playing "go fish" to low structured and low keyed discourse about an activity.

The clinician encouraged Adam to slow down his speech rate, because an increase in the amount of disfluency often occurred with rapid speech rate. Clinician modeling of "soft" slow-normal speech with easy onset continued to be used.

● *Sessions 10 to 18*   Analogies to "easy" versus "hard" speech were made first by the clinician simulating "easy" (soft, less tense) and "hard" (loud, tense, forced) animal sounds such as a cat's "meow" or a dog's bark. The technique served two purposes: first, as a transition to Adam's differentiating "easy" from "hard" manner of speaking in his own speech (he continued to be somewhat wary when directly approached about his own stuttering), and second because examining animal sounds is less abstract to a 4-year-old than analyzing one's own speech. By session 18, Adam demonstrated an understanding of "easy" and "hard" speech.

● *Sessions 19 to 26*   By this time, Adam and the clinician incorporated more specific types of disfluencies under the general term "hard speech" from Adam's own stuttering symptomatology. In fact, during Session 22, Adam himself identified rising pitch and prolongations ("holding the sound for a long time") as well as facial contortions as symptoms of stuttering. Fluency-enhancing techniques such as slower and smoother speech, lower volume and pitch, and simpler linguistic units continued to be used. The parents also had begun to notice an overall improvement in Adam—a calmer child, less stuttering at home, and less adverse attention paid to Adam's speech by parents and grandparents. Frequent conferences with Adam's mother facilitated these improvements. However, the mother reported that keeping the general level of activity down when the two boys were together continued to be difficult. We found the mother to be a pivotal and indispensable ally in providing insights about the home environment and in helping Adam to implement some of the therapy objectives at home when generalization activities were initiated.

● *Sessions 34 to dismissal (after three semesters of therapy)*   By the thirty-fourth session, Adam exhibited less than 1% syllables stuttered during a language sample taken. Most of the disfluencies occurred on pronouns and verbs. Session 36 started a third and final semester at our clinic. Adam maintained his high rate of fluency over the winter break, so that the primary goals for the third semester included maintaining fluency in increasingly more complex linguistic contexts, as well as varying the pragmatic functions of Adam's discourse. We found that his associated symptoms rescinded without need for formal therapy, as the core symptoms subsided.

However, as Adam's utterances and the ideas he attempted to convey became more complex, he tended to increase the rate of speaking and to use run-on sentences. Moreover, his breathing pattern during the run-on sentences became somewhat discoordinated. Whenever this was observed, the clinician simply asked Adam to "Tell the story a little at a time." At one point, when he was experiencing greater than usual amounts of disfluency because of the heightened linguistic load, Adam said to the clinician, "I have to think first." Various everyday situations were simulated in the therapy sessions for generalization of fluency behavior. Pragmatic considerations were added to the therapy. That is, Adam was asked to consider the listener's viewpoint when he was talking about an event that was convoluted and more vulnerable to disfluencies. The idea of giving the listener "a chance to follow the story" by watching the listener's face for feedback was successfully initiated during Session 51.

Followup   Generalization of fluency to situations and persons outside the therapy context (e.g., other buildings on campus, situations at home) continued. Before dismissal, Adams's younger brother was invited to join the sessions. In addition to improvement in fluency, Adam also exhibited slower speech rate, fewer run-on sentences, and very appropriate and skillful use of pragmatics. The family was ready to embark on a summer trip abroad to visit the paternal grandparents and other relatives. Followup interviews were scheduled for after the trip to Italy to ensure Adam's maintenance of fluency.

REFERENCES

Adams, M. R. 1980. The young stutterer: Diagnosis, treatment and assessment of progress. Semin. Speech Lang. Hear. 1:289–300.

Ainsworth, S. H. 1977. If Your Child Stutters: A Guide for Parents. Speech Foundation of America, Memphis.

Bloodstein, O. 1981. A Handbook on Stuttering. 3rd Ed. National Easter Seal Society, Chicago.

Bloom, L., and Lahey, M. 1978. Language Development and Disorders. John Wiley & Sons, New York.

Borden, G. J., and Harris, K. S. 1980. Speech Science Primer: Physiology, Acoustics, and Perception of Speech. William & Wilkins Company, Baltimore.

Conture, E. G. 1982. Stuttering. Prentice-Hall, Englewood Cliffs, N. J.

Douglass, E., and Quarrington, B. 1952. The differentiation of interiorized and exteriorized secondary stuttering. J. Speech Hear. Disord. 17:377–385.

Ginott, H. G. 1965. Between Parent and Child: New Solutions to Old Problems. Macmillan Company, New York.

Gregory, H. H., and Hill, D. 1980. Stuttering therapy for children. Semin. Speech Lang. Hear. 1:351–363.

Guitar, B., and Peters, T. J. 1980. Stuttering: An Integration of Contemporary Therapies. Speech Foundation of America, Memphis.

Guitar, B., Kopfs, H., Kilbourg, G., and Conway, P. 1981. Parent verbal interactions and speech rate: A case study in stuttering. Paper presented at the American Speech-Language-Hearing Association Convention, Los Angeles.

Kline, M. L., and Starkweather, C. W. 1979. Receptive and expressive language performance in young stutterers. Paper presented at the American Speech-Language-Hearing Association Convention, Atlanta.

Luper, H. L., and Mulder, R. L. 1964. Stuttering: Therapy for Children. Prentice-Hall, Englewood Cliffs, N. J.

Mowrer, D. E. 1979. A Program to Establish Fluent Speech. Charles E. Merrill Publishers, Columbus, Ohio.

Nelson, L. A. 1982. Evaluation of disfluency, prevention of stuttering, and management of fluency problems in children. Paper presented at the conference sponsored by the Speech Foundation of America, Chicago.

Nelson, N. W. 1979. Planning Individualized Speech and Language Intervention Programs. Communication Skill Builders, Tuscon.

Riley, G., and Riley, J. 1979. A component model for diagnosing and treating children who stutter. J. Fluency Disord. 4:279–293.

Riley, G. D., and Riley, J. 1980. Motoric and linguistic variables among children who stutter: A factor analysis. J. Speech Hear. Disord. 45:504–514.

Ryan, B. P. 1979. Stuttering therapy in a framework of operant conditioning and programmed learning. In: H. H. Gregory (ed.), Controversies About Stuttering Therapy, pp. 129–173. University Park Press, Baltimore.

Ryan, B., and Van Kirk, B. 1978. Monterey Fluency Program. Monterey Learning Systems, Palo Alto, Calif.

Shine, R. E. 1980. Direct management of the beginning stutterer. Semin. Speech Lang. Hear. 1:339–350.

Silverman, F. H., and Williams, D. E. 1972. Prediction of stuttering by school-aged stutterers. J. Speech Hear. Res. 15:189–193.

Stocker, B. 1980. The Stocker Probe Technique: for Diagnosis and Treatment of Stuttering in Young Children. Modern Education Corporation, Tulsa.

Van Riper, C. 1971. The Nature of Stuttering. Prentice-Hall, Englewood Cliffs, N. J.

Van Riper, C. 1973. The Treatment of Stuttering. Prentice-Hall, Englewood Cliffs, N. J.

Van Riper, C. 1982. The Nature of Stuttering. 2nd Ed. Prentice-Hall, Englewood Cliffs, N. J.

Wall, M. J. 1980. A comparison of syntax in young stutterers and non-stutterers. J. Fluency Disord. 5:321–326.

Webster, R. L. 1979. Empirical considerations regarding stuttering therapy. In H. H. Gregory (ed.), Controversies About Stuttering Therapy. University Park Press, Baltimore.

Williams, D. 1971. Stuttering therapy for children. In: L. E. Travis (ed.), Handbook of Speech Pathology and Audiology, pp. 1073–1093. Appleton-Century-Crofts, New York.

Williams, D. 1979. A perspective on approaches to stuttering therapy, pp. 241–268. In H. H. Gregory (ed.), Controversies About Stuttering Therapy. University Park Press, Baltimore.

Index